BEEF

◆ THE UNTOLD STORY ◆

of How

Milk, Meat, and Muscle
Shaped the World

BEEF

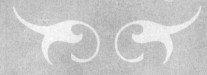

ANDREW RIMAS

◆ AND ◆

EVAN D. G. FRASER

wm

WILLIAM MORROW

An Imprint of HarperCollinsPublishers

Grateful acknowledgment is made for permission to reprint the following material: Excerpt on page 156 from "John Wayne: A Love Song" from *Slouching Towards Bethlehem* by Joan Didion, copyright 1966, 1968, renewed 1996 by Joan Didion. Reprinted by permission of Farrar, Straus and Giroux, LLC. Excerpt on page 197 from "The King's Breakfast" from *When We Were Very Young* by A. A. Milne, illustrations by E. H. Shepard, copyright 1924 by E. P. Dutton, renewed 1952 by A. A. Milne. Used by permission of Dutton Children's Books, A Division of Penguin Young Readers Group, A Member of Penguin Group (USA) Inc., 345 Hudson Street, New York, NY 10014. All rights reserved (US publisher). Excerpt on page 197 from "The King's Breakfast" from *When We Were Very Young* by A. A. Milne © The Trustees of the Milne estate. Published by Egmont UK Ltd. London and used with permission (UK publisher).

HarperCollins books may be purchased for educational, business, or sales promotional use. For information please write: Special Markets Department, HarperCollins Publishers, 10 East 53rd Street, New York, NY 10022.

FIRST INTERNATIONAL EDITION

Designed by Janet M. Evans

Library of Congress Cataloging-in-Publication Data

Rimas, Andrew.
    Beef : the untold story of how milk, meat, and muscle shaped the world / Andrew Rimas and Evan D. G. Fraser.—1st ed.
      p. cm.
    Includes bibliographical references and index.
    ISBN 978-0-06-135384-0
    1. Cattle—History.   I. Fraser, Evan D. G.   II. Title.

  SF195.R56 2008
  636.2009—dc22   2008002906

  ISBN 978-0-06-171879-3 (international edition)

08 09 10 11 12 ov/RRD 10 9 8 7 6 5 4 3 2 1

TO ANNINA, FYNN, AND SOPHIA

• CONTENTS •

· INTRODUCTION ·

If you shimmy a jeep down the Uplands Road that falls, like a stream of shattered asphalt, from Nairobi into the Great Rift Valley, you'll come to a broad green world that's full of cows.

You see them as you drop past the cascading trees and onto the tilled flats, passing cornfields, satellite dishes, and squat hamlets that blister up from the dust. Cows are everywhere. You see them alone on the roadside, strolling in sixes and dozens; grazing by the hundreds. Leaning on signs for the DELIVERANCE CHURCH and PARADISE HOTEL, staring mournfully at mosques and butcher shops. You see them in the foreground of brambling woods, while giraffes scud and tack above billows of wild sage. They speck distant pastures and brush against the side-door mirrors of your car. Everywhere, you see fixed brown eyes, muddy hooves, and shoulders rolling at a thoughtful plod. Everywhere, you see cattle.

It was here, about three million years ago, that human beings took one of their most resolute evolutionary steps. The Rift Valley is where a lithe, soft-furred hominid called *Australopithecus afarensis* loped and waddled for a short time until she turned into a significant fossil. This was humanity's common foremother, familiar today on account of a skull named Lucy. She would have known shade under the sage bushes, and hot dust and predators in the open grass. And, 2.5 million years ago, just like now, she would have known cows. Crouching in the acacias' thorny crooks, our ancestors looked on as horned giants scraped and lowed and thundered. Sometimes, these early hominids would find a carcass and scoop at the fat and purple muscle, licking at the blood. We evolved together, cows and us. We are old, old companions.

Driving through the valley today, you'll also see the people who own the cattle, the Masai. In the century and a half since the English arrived, this tiny, storied tribe has tried to ignore everything from nuclear fusion to Karen von Blixen: they still wear red shuka cloaks instead of trousers; they still distend their earlobes to a spaniel droop. To the Masai, the Iron Age has never lost its allure. And they still live for cattle—herding them, milking them, counting them, fighting over them, and comparing them for size. Mostly, though, they just watch them. There isn't a cowboy or gaucho in the world who understands cattle better than does a four-year-old Masai.

Our first glimpse of the valley was through the fly-speckled windshield of a jeep that careened like a sprinting drunk between ruts deep enough to crack an axle. We were late in getting to the village of Endikirt Osenyai, and our driver, a Masai named Jerry Ole Kina, wanted to reach it before sundown. Jerry is a big man among the Masai, quite literally since he tops six feet, all chest and shoulder and jawbone. As a veterinarian, he is something of a celebrity in a tribe that believes God gave them possession of all the cattle in the world. It's a peculiarity of the Masai that, out of all of Africa's treasures in gold and diamonds and fertile earth, they chose cows to carry the stamp of divine grace.

"They say that God gave the Masai cattle," said Jerry in that particular African timbre that sounds roasted like coffee. "They say it makes us different from the Kikuyu, with their seeds and hoes, or the Dorobo, with their bows and honeybees. And it makes us different from the white man, with his books."

That's what they say.

They're wrong, of course. For ten thousand years, people in Africa, Europe, and Asia have claimed dominion over cattle, very often over the herds that belong to their neighbors. Coveting cows is an ancient vice, and their theft, if not the most timeworn style of wickedness, is as old as Cain. Cows have always roused our acquisitive instincts. The first reason for this is also the one that's the most animal.

◆ How *to* Eat Beef ◆

The most profligate dish on the menu at the Grill 23 restaurant in Boston—and this is a menu carbuncled with oysters—is the Berkeley. Weighing, like a slice off a prizefighter, at an exact sixteen ounces and hung to dry for two to four weeks to let its juices brew, it's the sort of rib eye steak that people order at birthdays or coronations. As moist as a melon, its filaments cleave at the glimmer of a knife. Seared but not blackened, the middle is salmon pink darkening to a clean streak of lobster red, with a taste that's not too marrowy, but that's touched with nuts and greens; the fat runs clear. The cow from which it's harvested is the Dutch Frisian, a dairy animal fed on flaked corn, alfalfa, and Sudan grass, and its silky flavor is unusual to a palate accustomed to rough Black Angus. This meat needs no sauce, no pepper, and no clever dressing. An accompanying clod of spinach creamed with cheese and bacon is as unnecessary as the fat potato on the edge of the plate. As far as a dinner entrée can be both vainglorious and refined, this is.

Herodotus thought that history began with rape, with the tit-for-tat abductions of Io, Europa, Medea, and then the final, unforgivable business of Helen. He was wrong. History isn't the story of sex. It's the story of food. The Berkeley is why people have always collected cows. Human beings love beef. They love its perfumed smoke, they love its roiling drops of blood and grease, they love its density, so much more gravid in the belly than any vegetable, like ballast for living. Most of all, human beings love its panoply of flavors. A single cut of sirloin can taste liverish and sweet. Veal is milky. Chuck is dark, lush, even earthy like an opulent wine.

To be meaty means to possess merit and conviction. To be vegetal means to be practically dead.

There are vegetarians at large in America today who, when asked if they ever felt a carnivorous tug, mumble something about childhood. "I ate a lot of beef when I was a kid" is a typical response. "Hamburgers and hot dogs and bologna, that sort of thing. But then it stopped tasting good."

These vegetarians are right. Beef today tastes drab compared with the T-bones of yore. A generation ago, beef had a more vigorous snap in its juices. Its loin cuts tasted more sugary, its flatiron steak more gamey. Everything from lowly burger meat to the juicy tip of the top sirloin (once called the honeymoon roast) was nearer the Platonic ideal. This isn't nostalgia for a lost world of Main Street butchers and window-dressed chops roosting, like scarlet birds, in parsley. The unhappy truth is that beef today is different because cattle today are different. They eat different food. Their bloodstreams pulse with different medicines. It's obvious why so many dejected beef eaters, fearing cholesterol, trans fats, water pollution, veal crates, hormone injections, *E. coli,* and mad cow scares, threw up their hands (and luncheon meats) and switched to trout.

"For years, I didn't eat meat," says Jay Murray, the executive chef at Grill 23 and the man who cooks the Berkeley rib eye. "I didn't think that beef had much flavor."

Not all of it does. Cattle aren't created equal, and their differences widen with age. As a rule, younger, fattier meat is perceived to have the best taste. "Meat science" uses numerical data like skeletal maturity, preliminary yield grades, and marbling subunits to calculate the expected tenderness of a carcass, and hence its worth. There's art involved, as well as science. The U.S. Department of Agriculture awards grades to beef, much like figure-skating judges rank a lutz. Inspectors eye the marbling (flecks of fat within the lean part of the meat) and stamp the beef with a grade: Prime, Choice, Select, Standard, Commercial, Utility, Cutter, or Canner. Prime makes up a mere 3 percent of graded beef and is usually sold exclusively to steakhouses—fodder for the rich. Choice is what you buy in supermarkets, as is Select, which is a shade tougher. Standard and Commercial are stringy enough to be "ungraded" and only appear masked under brand-name plastic. The rest is the stuff of frankfurters.

But these grades, while useful, only hint at the yawning chasm between the merely edible and the glorious.

"Cattle are like Xerox copies," says Murray. "They've faded. Through crossbreeding, we've lost the flavor."

The cows we eat in America today are mostly descended from long, muddy tributaries of the British Hereford (both Horned and Polled) and Angus (Red and Black), and the Continental breeds like Charolais, Limousin, and Simmental. Crossbreeding has "improved" them, made them productive in the manner of sprouting fast from calf to giant carcass, but it's also made them less tasty. From their British family, the cows inherited an ability to give birth with slippery ease. Continental relatives gave them size and leanness. As a result of crossbreeding, American cattle today are whalelike creatures encased, not in blubber, but in red, salable meat. The problem is that it's so insipid. And even the pure breed meat like Angus isn't always the most flavorful.

"Butchers like Angus because the carcass yields are so high," says Murray. "But when you look at the steaks, the familiar white lines of the marbling don't eat well. There's no consistency. It's fat followed by toughness, followed by fat." As a rule, Americans prize texture above flavor. The most popular dish at steakhouses is tenderloin—filet mignon—both for its name recognition and for its suppleness, but not for its richness or character. You need a rib eye for that.

ᘓ ᘔ

CULINARY INTERLUDE

Rib Eye Steak

According to Grill 23's executive chef Jay Murray, the king of beef is the rib eye steak. Meat from the shoulder blade (terras major) can challenge tenderloin for texture, while boasting a more concentrated flavor. The top blade or flatiron is gamey and soft—if you close your eyes while eating it, you might mistake it for duck. Lean tri-tip steak, also called sirloin tip, has a full, complex flavor, and if not overcooked (Brazilians salt it for two hours, then grill it rare) can rival any chop on the carcass.

But it's six bones down the rib cage, at the vertebral end of the ribs, that you'll find a steak that has the largest proportion of long dorsal muscle (longissimus dorsi). This rib eye is the most perfect piece of meat on a cow.

Jay Murray's recipe for a 1¼-inch rib eye steak is simple, verging on spartan. Sear the meat with butter in a heavy skillet. Flip after two minutes, then fry for another sixty seconds. "Searing changes the nature of the proteins on the edges, adding a ton of flavor." Place the browned meat under the broiler for another six minutes to finish it. If the steak is of high-enough quality, the only seasoning needed is a brush of butter mixed with a few dabs of Worcestershire sauce.

Spartan in simplicity, yes, but the result should debauch the staunchest vegan.

Sauces on steak are a controversy. Latin recipes favor acidic ones like Argentine chimichurri—a mash of parsley, garlic, olive oil, salt, and pepper—that contrast with the richness of the beef. French sauces are the opposite. They rely on reductions of stock, cognac, or red wine to augment the meat's natural flavor, or on emulsions of butter and egg yolk like béarnaise sauce to smother it.

Purists, of course, use none of them. Good meat is enough in itself. If you want tarragon and shallots, order a salad.

Once roasts are introduced into the discussion, however, the rules change. Roasts, lacking the caramelized surface area of steaks, have a softer flavor that profits from dressing, and flank steak is absurd unless it's steeped in something. Roasts have the spirit of the trestle, noise and communion, children, spilled gravy, and Grandmother's china. Steak is less familial. It's private and greedy, even intemperate; a surfeit of hoarded delight. Steak isn't a sin necessarily, but it's best when it feels like one.

◆ Big Trouble *in the* Beef Business ◆

There's no sense in arguing about how to sauce a good sirloin if a good sirloin can't be bought. The beef industry, like American agriculture as a whole, is entering a brave new world of price gouging, water shortages, diseased product, environmental collapse, and hyperactive markets. Dairy is no different. There's an irony in the fact that plenty has never been so plentiful, yet supply so fragile at the root. This isn't apparent from glancing at industry forecasts or at the contents of shopping carts. Market price, consumer demand, and many economic barometers make for chipper reading. Today, we pay less for rump steak, Brie, gelato, or low-fat yogurt than we've done at any point in history, and we eat more of it. Our cows are gigantic and healthy (if health can be measured in terms of production). Their bodies yield a purity of salable meat, wasting only shreds of fat and skin. In the United States, beef and dairy costs remain low enough so that, to misquote Herbert Hoover, we have a roast in every pot and a cheese pizza in every microwave. Due in large part to our happy glut of cattle, we've swapped the specter of malnutrition for the wheezing ills of obesity, heart disease, and diabetes. It seems like a permanent trade.

But nothing in history is permanent, with the possible exception of a bad name, an echoing failure like Chernobyl, or a melting ice cap. There's a price to be paid for our cornucopia of flesh. Environmental wounds—waterways fouled by slurry, underground springs drained to irrigate crops wasted on animal feed—are the most apparent costs, but there are more insidious ones. Rising fuel costs are driving up the price of cattle feed, and in an industry stretched to thin financial margins, this can be disastrous. Diners are increasingly eyeing their meat for hormones and their milk for antibiotics. Mad cow proved that a fatal animal-borne disease seeping into our food chain isn't an oddity, but a growing likelihood. Even the seeming bargain of Our Daily Hamburger hides a high cost in taxes, since the cattle industry rests on the false props of subsidized fuel, government-funded agricultural research, and direct cash payments to farmers. Federal money, not market forces, is what keeps industrial cattle "factories" in operation. Were it not for government banknotes, cattle would exist on smaller farms, eating more grass than corn, and would fetch a steeper price once carved, wrapped, and scanned through the checkout register.

The cattle industry's troubles are leading to an inevitable conclusion: beef and milk are going to become more expensive. Aggressively so. We're coming to the climax of all our millennia of experiments in breeding cattle, in molding the landscape to feed them, and in enjoying the bounty of their flesh, milk, and muscle. This climax is the culmination of cattle themselves. Not as a species—as long as there's a commodity involved, we'll have creatures approximating cows. But they're not going to be the animals that evolved with us and shaped our civilization. They'll be strings of genes, meticulously plotted for the cheapest yield of product. They'll hardly be animals at all.

This is the story of cattle and of the people who made them what they are. It's a cautionary tale, but it doesn't have an ending yet. At least, not one that's fixed. Throughout the world, countless cattle owners treat their land and animals with a reverence far more sincere than the weekend platitudes of casual environmentalists, and many of them are finding ways to meld ancient husbandry with modern markets. But they're still too few in number.

There's still world enough, and time. But not much of either.

AUDUMLA

Then said Gangleri: "Where dwelt Ymir, or
wherein did he find sustenance?" Hárr answered:
"Straightway after the rime dripped, there sprang
from it the cow called Audumla; four streams of
milk ran from her udders, and she nourished
Ymir." Then asked Gangleri: "Wherewithal was the
cow nourished?" And Hárr made answer: "She
licked the ice-blocks, which were salty; and the first
day that she licked the blocks, there came forth
from the blocks in the evening a man's hair; the
second day, a man's head; the third day the whole
man was there."

—ON THE NORSE CREATION MYTH,
FROM *THE PROSE EDDA*

The central actor of the Viking creation myth is not a god, but a cow. Audumla licked life out of ice and nurtured it with her milk, an obvious thing for a cosmic cow to do in the minds of people whose survival depended on daily milk and a strong, bovine back to lug a plow. The first part of our story introduces us to ancient cattle and shows how we turned them into the milk, meat, and muscle on which we built civilization.

1

FROM HORN to HOOF

*The Ecological and Evolutionary
Origins of the Cow:
Prehistory–8000 B.C.*

♦ The Thread *in the* Labyrinth ♦
Picasso's Minotaur *and the* Spirit *of* Cattle

The Spanish pavilion at the 1937 Paris World's Fair opened to a puff of tepid headlines and a yawn from the summer-slow picnickers on the Seine. And no surprise. A few weeks earlier, Paris had weathered the openings of the Nazi German and Soviet pavilions—Herculean mounds of concrete erected to dueling ideologies, between which the modest Spanish building was a mere bungalow rolled out in the name of a lowercase "republicanism." Even the promised unveiling of a giant Picasso mural didn't stir up much more than froth in the café gossip.

That is, until people actually saw *Guernica*, as Picasso's painting is known. Its subject was an average atrocity by modern standards, but in 1937 it had the power to appall. Two months before the Paris exhibition, German bombers flying for the fascist side in the Spanish Civil

War obliterated a civilian target far from the front lines. The massacre killed fifteen hundred people. Picasso had long ago proven he could make strong critics faint and send belle artistes dashing for their fractured mirrors, but he had never yet managed to horrify everybody. It took *Guernica,* and Guernica, to do that.

The painting wasn't horrible because it depicted war. It was horrible for depicting horror. A twenty-three-foot slash of newsprint-colored violence, it hung behind a working fountain of red mercury. To Paris's lunching gentlemen and girls in frocks, this was something entirely new. Otto Dix and George Grosz had drawn the First World War's seas of corpses in the 1920s, but *Guernica*'s subject wasn't dead soldiers. It was women, children, and beasts in the act of dismemberment—limbs and heads separating by means of high explosives (making it a perfect subject for cubism, for Picasso's famous splintered eye). Gray and sickly, like a bruise the size of a whale, *Guernica* is a particularly modern obscenity. It's now an icon of the age of broken glass, airplanes, and random blood pools. Of the age that is our own.

Inside the picture itself, among the blasted innocents, stand two animals. One is a skewered horse, screaming in the dumb, brute pain of dying. The other is a bull standing under a lightbulb, its horns bulging from an asymmetrical skull lump that echoes its scrotal bag. The bull is a fixed hulk, unmoved by the slaughter around it. It may even be complicit, since the horse looks like it's been gored. During an interview in 1944, Picasso said that the bull represented "dark forces," while the horse stood for the Spanish people. Another time he insisted, exasperatedly, that "The bull is a bull and the horse is a horse. These are openly animals, massacred animals. That's all, so far as I am concerned!"[1]

Well, no. Picasso didn't like to give away his metaphors, and a bull, especially one placed by a Spanish painter inside his greatest work, isn't mere bystanding livestock. A bull is always more than that. Is it Picasso's original "dark forces"? Distilled cruelty? The animal mask of war? Or is it a symbol for the Spanish nation?[2]

Good art, much less great art, isn't a code, like a peach clutched by some dusty medieval Virgin. To grope for an exclusive truth behind Picasso's bull misses the point that bulls, like lions, eagles, and unicorns, are charged with millennia of cultural presumptions. So while we can argue that the bull represents Spain, and its stillness is a counterpoint to the screeching female stumbling up from the lower right-hand field, thereby hinting at a dichotomy more elemental than mere political symbols, that would be playing the game of allegories.[3] The *Guernica* bull isn't a national totem, nor is it shorthand for brutality. It's bigger than that.

Picasso understood that the bull, beyond its heraldic clutter, is a throwback to a time before cities existed to be bombed, before civilization existed to be shocked. Under the glare of an electric bulb, we see an ancient face that is neither good nor evil. It is solely dangerous.

Painters all have their favorite monsters, and Picasso's was the Minotaur, the man-bull that crouches, steeped in a Freudian fog, at the center of the artist's twists and feints. Picasso hammered out Minotaurs like a refrain.[4] He drew them attacking women, or raising a glass to toast the spent bodies in an orgy, or being held at bay by the frail light of a child's upheld candle. They are dark forces, masculine ones. In one etching from 1934, a blind Minotaur walks hand in hand with a girl clutching a plump, white dove—dark forces tamed. But that was before the German bombers flew their devilish sorties over a living city in the north of Spain, leading Picasso to paint a bull that stands, unflinching, in the jagged nexus between primeval force and the phosphorus bomb.

The paradox of *Guernica*'s bull is that it exists in two worlds, an ancient creature bathed in an antiseptic, high-wattage glow. Bulls have become beasts of the stockyard and the chemical feed trough, but their bodies are testaments to long-vanished grasslands and unmarred skies. To understand the spirit that infuses Picasso's painting you have to look at history—a maze more tangled than the logical weave of silicon circuits. This is history as a labyrinth; by turn and corner, this has to be felt to be explored. Artists are naturals at doing this, and Picasso, in the electric dawn of the Jaded Age, was the great artist of his time, proving his mastery by showing the Paris crowds that, despite our newfound knack with motors and steel, we are no different from our grandsires who scraped at flint in the starlight. The story behind the *Guernica* bull must begin with its flesh, its meat, and its horn.

In Picasso's Spain, bulls lived both in bleached concrete pens and in an ancient place of symbols, sun, and blood. They still do today. Spain is where the thread leads into the labyrinth.

The little farm of "Las Mojadillas" sits in the hills off the Merida highway running south from Seville. The nearest villages are ramshackle clusters of worn plaster and scaffolded churches, running to decay due more to a lack of urgency than to a lack of funds. But a traveler's eye would skip them anyway, for they're buried in a swathe of *encinas* and holm oaks, the gnarled, flint-barked trees that stoop like sheltering grandmothers over the entirety of southern Spain. The farmhouse itself looks like a villa built by the ancient Romans who used to raise cattle in these parts. Two white and yellow stories hooked around a yard parked with horses, red tiles above, swept cobbles below, prettied by dabs of ceramic and terra-cotta.

The proprietor of Las Mojadillas is Pedro Trapote, supplier of prime fighting bulls to the Spanish arena. It's an old profession, imprinted with memories (some false) of the Roman amphitheater and the American rodeo. Wearing a neat flannel shirt and pressed jeans, Trapote, who has black hair as dense as a schnauzer's, is the image of a Spanish gentleman farmer, down to the frantic cell phone and undying Marlboro.

"The bull represents force, brute strength," says Trapote, himself a masculine entity, perhaps because his dark eyes pulse with the burn from a two-day whisky bender. "But it also is a philosopher of the field. It is the noblest animal."

He's right, in the definition of nobility as rare blood. On the wall of the villa's central courtyard, like a shrine to the house's guardian ancestors, sprouts a tiled family tree painted, not with upstanding Trapotes, but with each branch and shoot of the bulls' expensive lineage. This dates back a century, but the farmland on which the bulls live is much older. It's a weathered quilt of oaks mixed with olives, pale grass, and tumbled stones.

"It takes three hundred years to lay the foundations for a farm like this," says Trapote, casting a hand across the swells of earth. Or longer. Cattle have run here since the ice first unveiled these hills to the Mediterranean sun. *Toros bravos* is the name the Spanish give to these cows, an atavistic race that bridges the Neolithic and popular television shows. Bullfighting, regardless of the cries of animal rights groups, is a link in a cultural chain stretching back to prehistory.

We saw our first toro bravo lying in the northern lee of a holm oak, as calm as a spinster at her knitting. She was an elderly cow, perhaps eight years old, delicate and brown, her cool, pooling eyes fixed on the gnats. Her udder was unobtrusive, not inflated like that of a Holstein, and she wore her stubby horns brushed up, like a giraffe's. She hardly looked like the mother of furies. Across the farm, past Trapote's villa and a miniature bullfighting arena, her sons brooded in the shade like idling tanks.

Fighting bulls are colored every hue from midnight black to speckled red to white, but Trapote's breed favors a conservative, solid chestnut. Their horns ideally jut laterally from the skull, then curve forward, then up.[5] Heads are large, and shoulders are hugely muscled, much as they should be in prizefighters. Trapote's one-year-olds pasture separately from the two-year-olds, who live apart from the three-year-olds, who themselves never see the arrogant four-year-old toros marked for the great bullfighting arenas in Madrid, Ronda, and Seville. Each bull is accorded an average of two to three hectares of wooded range on which to graze, run, and frolic its 600-kilogram bulk. Las Mojadillas bulls are considered slight. The giant Mihuras breed breaks the scale at 700 kilos, more or less equal to a "high-productivity" beef steer in the United States. The difference, of course, is that beef cows swell up in a very short time on high-calorie feed, antibiotics, and, in the United States, growth hormones. Toros bravos live like their ancestors on a

diet of wild grass, hay, and acorns, filled out during the winter by locally grown organic grass that's been cut and dried for use during the
colder weather. Until they enter the ring at the age of four, they're as
cosseted as orchids.

It's in the ring that the bulls leave behind the tang of the farmyard
and, like Picasso's Minotaurs, assume a larger meaning. One of these
rings is in San Sebastian de los Reyes, a blue-collar suburb of Madrid.
"Sanse," as it's called, is a graceless village, all concrete, graffiti, and
satellite dishes. The bullring is a colorless slab gassed by fumes from
the town's main bus stop. But what happens there on August mornings
has been going on in Spain since long before the birth of Christ.

At about 6:30 A.M., the men and boys, dressed in white and red,
gather in the oily streets around the Calle Real. They smoke and stare
at the pavement, still cool from the nighttime damp. Some of them sit
on wooden fences that have been raised along the sidewalks, while
mothers and wives dawdle in the doors of fluorescent cafés, looking at
their watches and laughing without smiling. Red and white are the
colors of sacrifice.

At a few minutes past seven, a firecracker bursts like a mortar and
shocks the town into silence. Then everyone inhales as two, then three
mad-eyed children sprint down the street toward the bullring. More
runners—girls and teenagers—giggling with fear. Minutes pass before
a low, grinding rumble shakes the fences, and the runners, who were
earlier merely sprinting, careen around the corner in a mass of whip-
ping torsos. Puny, with eyes like saucers, they're swept along by a wave
of giant backs and skulls of inhuman, rolling strength pushing at the
tips of knifing horns. The bulls are coming. God help us.

It's over in about fifteen seconds. The fallen are hauled up and
slapped around the shoulders, knees are dusted, chatter flows, and the
bulls disappear into the arena, where they're hidden until slaughter
that afternoon in front of a stadium crowd. As an addendum, the festival organizers release a few calves and small bullocks into the ring,
where the boldest teenagers dodge and vault the animals, risking a
minor goring for the cheers of the miniskirted girls in the bleachers.

Mediterranean youths have been reenacting this ritual for perhaps five thousand years.

The suburban Spanish teenager who splits his blue jeans while trying to hop over a bullock is part of a continuum. It merges Trapote's farm with the palaces of ancient Crete and the prairies of Paleolithic France. Toros bravos are the living face of that continuum. For millennia, we have painted, corralled, stolen, worshipped, slaughtered, and eaten the flesh of these muscled giants. We've leveled forests and raised temples for them. Civilizations have arisen on their backs and been fed on their milk. We've sculpted their genetics. And all those years, they've been changing us, too. Imagine our world without cattle, and you're not imagining our world. Cattle, second only to the ingenuity of humanity itself, built this astounding complexity of fields and cities, letters and money, banks and kings. And, indeed, of gods.

◆ What *Is a* Cow? ◆

Early on the sixth day of Creation, God said, "Let the earth bring forth the living creature after his kind, cattle, and creeping thing, and beast of the earth."[6] Later that afternoon, God took a stab at self-portraiture and made Man. From this we're to understand that animals, and cattle specifically, are our Sixth Day brethren. Note, however, the distinction made between cattle and "beasts of the earth." Cattle are actually beasts of the grass.

A cow is in every way a creature that lives for, on, and because of simple grass: a growth so mundane that, to most people, it registers less as a plant than as a style of carpeting. Cattle evolved to take advantage of grass species that became established during the temperate climates of the middle parts of the world during the Miocene epoch, about twenty-three million years ago. To a cow, grass is the alpha and omega. It's practically the entire palette of experience. The cow creation myth would begin, not with light, but with dew on the morning lawn.

Our own creation myths occasionally begin with cows. The Vikings told a story about Audumla, a cosmic bovine that suckled Ymir, the "rime-giant" whose sweat was so fertile that it begat the races of the Earth. According to Snorri Sturluson's *Prose Edda* (the Viking equivalent of the Old Testament): "Straightway after the rime dripped [from the primordial ice], there sprang from it the cow called Audumla; four streams of milk ran from her udders, and she nourished Ymir."

Audumla, being a cow, liked salt. This predilection gave birth to the first god:

> She licked the ice-blocks, which were salty; and the first
> day that she licked the blocks, there came forth from
> the blocks in the evening a man's hair; the second day,
> a man's head; the third day the whole man was there.
> He was named Búri: he was fair of feature, great and
> mighty.

Búri was the grandfather of Odin, the greatest of the gods, and one of his early accomplishments was to murder Ymir the milk drinker. The giant's corpse was so unfathomably gargantuan that Odin and his brothers pulped his flesh to make the earth, flooded the ocean basins with his blood, and cracked his bones to raise the mountainsides. The earth was made from the body of a milk drinker. It's hard to imagine a better advertisement for the nutritional and developmental properties of cows' milk.

Vikings, as well as giants, were a dairy-fed folk. They ferried cows (and a single, obstreperous bull) on their ships as far as North America, and we know that Viking settlers introduced cows' milk to the "Skraeling" natives they met, most likely the Beothuk tribe of Newfoundland. In exchange for precious furs and "the contents of [the natives'] packs," Viking women carried buckets of milk out to the gleeful Indians, who downed the contents while sitting on the ground outside the Norse encampment. It was a peaceable enough beginning for transatlantic relations. For several years, contact between the Europeans and the Americans consisted solely of exchanging furs for milk. Alas, it was inevitable that the traders began to argue, then to steal. And then to kill. The cows returned to Greenland with the last Viking ships, and Americans had to wait another five hundred years to again taste milk from a cow.

The Viking colony failed, but the animals that they brought to Newfoundland would have been very happy in their immigrant home. L'Anse aux Meadows is the modern name of the windswept headland where they settled; it's a chilly welter of salt bogs and scraggly forests called tuckamore by Newfoundlanders. There's a particularly northern joy, in summer, to stand there, on the sea-green sedge, and watch icebergs fleck the indigo horizon.

The cattle would have paid little attention to seascapes, though. They were concerned with something much more pressing, because, in addition to the mosses and liverwort that thrive in the briny air, L'Anse aux Meadows is home to ninety species of edible grass. This is all very exciting to a cow, for unless she spends the larger part of her waking hours in eating, she will die. From a biological perspective, cattle are Nature's lawn mowers—over millions of years they won their Darwinian battles through perfecting the trick of digesting grass, and they're suited to do little else.

Here's how. A cow's cheek teeth are hypsodont—with high crowns that extend above the gumline, leaving room for wear over long years of grinding—and selenodont—with ridges for breaking up stringy greens. The jaws work in circular motion, ideal for milling the hard fibers, after which the cow swallows its food into the first two chambers of its stomach, called the reticulorumen. Unlike in the human stomach, there are no corrosive gastric juices here. The animal's natural enzymes are not robust enough to break down coarse grass. So, the work of turning grass into nourishment has to be done by a wash of microbes that live in harmony within the cow's gut. After the cow digests its grass for a time, it sucks the pulp—called the cud—back into its gullet, gags it up into its mouth, tongues it against its palate to squish out the excess water, chews it a bit more, and swallows it back. Extra chewing has the effect of increasing the surface area onto which bacteria may latch. Chewing also has the side effect of stimulating the saliva glands. Spit buffers the cow's stomach acidity; if the cow stops chewing foraged plants, its rumen's acidity rises, lowering appetite. This leads to less chewing, which in turn cycles downward to less appetite. Eventually, the cow's metabolism collapses and it dies. Eat to live, indeed.

Once the cud is sufficiently deliquesced, it moves into the cow's third chamber, the omasum. This absorbs more water and nutrients before the food oozes into the abomasum, where the cow's digestive juices finally do their deconstructive work. The most significant of these enzymes is rennet, the active ingredient in cheese making.

All this chewing and swallowing occupies the cow for six to eight of its waking hours each day—cattle, like hedgehogs, are born specialists. The ruminant system also has the effect of keeping the cow vigorously flatulent at both ends of its digestive tract. The earth's ruminant livestock pass eighty million metric tons of methane gas per year—a gas also formed in oceans, rice paddies, and termite mounds.[7] The impact of bovine belching is, of course, awful. All this methane is a dangerous thickener in the atmosphere's soup of greenhouse gases—cows are much at fault for climate change, just as we are at fault for cows.

Pollution notwithstanding, the cow's stomach is remarkably good at digesting rough cellulose through the offices of successive, fermenting blasts of bacteria. It really is a triumph of evolution. Our human stomach is woefully prone to upset, being unable to grind the nutrients out of most greenery: we are monogastric, sharing a paltry one-chambered stomach with other omnivores like pigs and bears. The vegetarian ruminant, however, uses four chambers to convert some of the least nutritious parts of the plant world into a buffet. Imagine the sight of a verdant pasture, flush with clover. Now imagine that, like in Willy Wonka's Chocolate Factory, everything you see is sweet and edible—that almost the whole of creation can be experienced through the tongue. In such a world, to stand in a damp meadow would be more than bliss. It would be symphonic, an overwhelming delight beside which a human's brief, disjointed mealtimes must be thin pleasure. Grazing, to a cow, is not mere eating. It's the definition of life.

The cow's digestion isn't the only part of the animal that evolved for grazing. Its senses, too, suit it for eating grass. To better espy hunters (human or otherwise), a cow's eyes are wide apart on the sides of its head, according it wide-angle vision with a blind spot directly behind, a dim patch directly in front, and a keen alertness for movement. At the peripheries, images bend and, because cows have no sensitivity to color, the predator creeping at the flanks of the herd would appear as nothing more than a drab, twisted menace. To a cow, the grass is never greener, only darker. Shadows are entirely horrible. They look like holes to be sidestepped, while a ray of bright light sets off a welter of frightening contrasts.

The cow's natural timidity is exacerbated by its delicate hearing and smell. Any untoward noise is a reason to spook—contrary to the popular image of the whooping cowboy, cattlemen tend to speak in low tones for fear of alarming their animals. But the olfactory is the cow's organ of choice—not only for whiffing springtime sexual odors, but for recognizing family from foe, or for judging the distance of an errant calf. A cow snuffling the air is experiencing a flood of sensations that human beings can only visualize—we can imagine their complexity of experience only in terms of eyesight.

The cow's mind, too, is that of a grazer. A herd is a flowing mass that, on the ideal prairie, moves in a rough, round clump. Its leaders, however, are not the dominant animals. Like people, cattle are intimately concerned with hierarchy, but theirs is shaped less like a social pyramid than like an hourglass. The strongest, most willful animals stay in the center of the group, enjoying a sheltered placement, while the cattle that actually guide the herd's movements are comparative weaklings. Primacy is further exhibited in feeding. The strongest take the foremost, central place at a trough, with lesser beasts pushed to the edges, providing a bulwark against predators.

Herd formations are natural to many other species, including birds, fish, and bats. Unlucky "marginal" individuals are pushed to the periphery where they're subject to being picked off by hostile carnivores—it's a "selfish" geometry. According to evolutionary biologist

W. D. Hamilton, that's why cattle are social animals. On their own, cows are slump-necked naifs, staring at the ground with weak eyes, focused on nothing but their immediate dinner. A lone cow would be swallowed by the first opportunistic tiger that comes along. But a cow that gangs together with a friend would lower its risk of being eaten to a 50 percent probability—a tiger can only gobble one animal at a time. More cows lessen the risk proportionally, and also increase the chance that a predator will be noticed by a glance or snuffle. So herds accumulate for protection. Cows being no less egotistical than people, the strong push the weak to the peripheries, claiming the safest, central spot by right of brawn.[8]

There are happy exceptions. Bison, arguably the most high-minded of ungulates, face an attack by gathering around the frailest members of the herd. Like hoplites in a phalanx, they stand together, presenting a unified line of horn and shoulder outward to their foes. But biologists agree that most herds arrange themselves more selfishly, with the strong hiding behind a sacrificial line of the aged and infirm. An ironic effect is that the most successful herds, being the largest, end up attracting the most predators. So a large herd with lots of offspring will often splinter into two, the better to discourage hunters.[9]

つ☞

CULINARY INTERLUDE
Nine Primal Cuts

Cattle's most voracious predator has always been humankind. But because a solitary person is even more feeble than an individual cow, our ancestors bunched together in order to attack, outflank, and trap the huge beasts that made for the best eating. It's often been speculated that human language and community originated in this unending hunt for barbecue. Here, then, are nine plausible or "primal" reasons why human beings would have come together to hunt in groups, and to risk the deadly horns of their prey.

Reason One ‡ SHORT LOIN

Rich and flabby, this is the pampered king of all cuts, from which porterhouse and filet mignon descend. The meat is buttery and dense with juice, but not with filament. When cooked rare or medium, it splits at the whisper of a knife. Ordering it well done is gross vandalism.

Reason Two ‡ RIB

Rib eye steak is arguably more flavorful than the porterhouse due to its thick marbling of fat. It's almost as tender as the pricier loin, and most chefs prefer it for its stronger taste. For roasts, the standing rib cut is the pinnacle. Without needing so much as a scent of garlic or herbs, prime rib surpasses even lobster or caviar as an animal luxury.

Reason Three ‡ SIRLOIN

The most bourgeois of cuts, sirloin is taken from the lower part of the ribs. Banal flavor and miserly tenderness are compensated for by size and affordability. Overcooked, it's like eating a wallet. Rare and sauced with béarnaise, it blooms like a rose in sunlight.

Reason Four ‡ CHUCK

This proletarian meat makes up 28 percent of beef in the carcass. Harvested from the working muscles in the neck and shoulder, it can actually reach transcendence in the cross-rib pot roast, stewed in broth or wine or Guinness. The steaks have a rustic charm if marinated for a day, then broiled with shallots.

Reason Five ‡ BRISKET

The lower chest is the source of slow-cooked ethnic dishes like hickory barbecue and Irish corned beef. Heavy with cartilage, it requires tricks like smoke and brine to coax out its hidden beauties.

Reason Six ‡ PLATE

Tough yet fatty, this belly meat is best exemplified by skirt steak, which is useless without a marinade. When seasoned, grilled, and cut across the grain, it finds dignity, if not natural character.

Reason Seven ‡ FLANK

Another belly meat, flank is inedible without being soaked in wine, soy sauce, or fruit juice. It's the world's chief source for stir fries, as well as the overrated London broil.

Reason Eight ‡ ROUND

So lean and unyielding that it needs to be beaten into yielding a flavor, round steaks require braising in sauce or masking with batter.

Reason Nine ‡ SHANK

This is leg meat that's rarely sold in supermarkets. Its highest ambition is hamburger.

This nine-point butcher's list is a crassly reductive view of cattle, cutting everything down to serving size. It makes the altogether typical mistake of failing to see the herd for the short rib. If we step back in perspective, though, these nine cuts of meat, and the animal from which we harvest them, become a biological history book—a tale of humanity's journey from the Ice to the Digital Ages, told in bone and sinew and mitochondria. It is our own story.

◆ Domestication ◆
How *the* Cows Came Home

Like the myth of the Viking creation, the story of civilization and cattle begins with a giant. His name was *Bos primigenius*, and he was the wild aurochs, sometimes called the wisent. He was the strutting, bellowing grandfather of today's cattle, standing at about five-foot-seven (1.7 m) at the withers with saber-shaped, inward-curving horns. The aurochs stomped into human cultural history in the Paleolithic and left it in 1627, when the last specimen died, lamented, in central Poland.

The aurochs obsessed Stone Age hunters with its spirit, its strength, and its metric ton of raw steak. We know this because before the sun and moon, before the gods, the cow was the first subject of human art.

In the Lascaux caves, buried under France's green Dordogne hills, there's a chamber called the Great Hall of the Bulls. This dim crevice is where Paleolithic art reached its zenith. After seeing it, other cave artists must have thrown away their pig hair and twigs, their ochre palettes and lumps of hematite, and said, "That's what we were trying to do all along! That's the spirit we sought to capture. And now it's done!"

The bulls depicted on the walls of the cave are aurochs. Seventeen thousand years ago, early Frenchmen crept away from the wind and sun to paint them on the vaulted rock ceiling. *Paint* is perhaps less appropriate a word than *sculpt*. The figures meld into the natural contours of the chamber. They rear and gallop and collapse into one another's lines. They're at once naturalistic and cartoonish, blending odd perspectives and sizes with masterly muzzles, backs, and running legs. The aurochs—which appear fifty-two times in Lascaux, and one of which is eighteen feet long—practically thunder in the underground silence.[10] They don't run so much as fly through the rock. That's why these aurochs, as well as the paintings of tumbling bison at Altamira and the horned sorcerer of Les Trois-Frères, are deemed masterworks worthy of launching a thousand art history textbooks. They're humanity's first durable achievements.

The prehistorian Abbè Henri Breuil thought that these cave paintings held a magical function, a sympathetic purpose in helping hunters bring down game. Perhaps. Food has always been one of our biggest obsessions. But zoologist R. Dale Guthrie has argued that at least some of the paintings—including the far more numerous Paleolithic handprints, random lines and dots, and etchings of genitals and breasts—were possibly the work of teenage boys, daring each other to enter dark places and leave their marks. This would make the images less spiritual icons than graffiti, youthful energy spewed in ink. As anyone who's ever taken the time to read the wall of a toilet stall knows, graffiti is a snapshot of rudimentary wants and impulses. Whether art or graffiti, the paintings reveal what was on the surface of the Paleolithic mind: a powerful interest in bulls.

The Lascaux cave artists lived on what has been called "the Mammoth Steppe," a vast, arid plain, chilled by the continental ice that sprawled from Europe through Asia and the Bering Straits and into North America. As a cultural milieu, the Mammoth Steppe promoted a meat diet, open-air living, and the sort of egalitarianism we romanticize in stories about wagon trains and the open frontier. Hunter-gatherer groups never grew much larger than about forty strong. No one owned much, so no one had wealth to envy or to peddle into influence. Women nursed babies, worked leather, and kept camp. Men hunted. This left children to mess about in dark caves, imagining the animals that formed the basis of their diets, their ambitions, and their dreams.

Of these, the aurochs was one of the grandest. It probably evolved in India between 1.5 and 2 million years ago, after which it lumbered after forage across Europe, Africa, and Asia. During the colder climatic shifts of the Pleistocene, it could never match the ruggedness of mammoths, bison, horses, and woolly rhinos, and when the glaciers crept south, the aurochs hugged the Mediterranean. Nor did it ever spread as far as northern Scandinavia or Ireland. But for tens of thousands of years, Paleolithic hunters chased it, painted it, cut its skin into capes and shoes and tents, and ate it.

When the ice receded and the forests of today's Holocene epoch crept over the ancient steppe, the aurochs thrived in the damp, sprouting woodlands. The great bulls roamed the sedge along rivers blistering with geese and ducks, feeding on the long marsh grasses, rutting in the late summer and birthing in the spring; their habitat wouldn't have been dissimilar to that of the modern moose. Cows herded separately from grown bulls, for good reason. Bulls were violent. When they met along a grazing track or across the scent of a cow, they dueled, slashing with their horns and tearing up the earth. We'll never have the privilege of seeing an aurochs battle again, but the clashes were so terrific that their tempers were proverbial until modern times.[11] Eyewitness descriptions of aurochs tended to be a little breathless. Even Julius Caesar, who doesn't pause much to admire the fauna on his campaigns, thought enough of the Gallic aurochs to say: "[They are] a little below the elephant in size, and of the appearance, color, and the shape of a bull. Their strength and speed are extraordinary; they spare neither man nor wild beast which they have espied."[12]

To imagine an aurochs battle, we really need the assistance of poetry. Although literature about the subject is sparse, we can get a measure of the beasts' ferocity from an ancient verse describing warring bulls. In this line from an Irish epic, a magical bull named the Donn Cúailnge has just rampaged across the island fighting his mortal enemy, the bull Findbennach Aí. He's just won:

> He raised his head haughtily and shook the remains
> of the Whitehorned from him over Erin. He sent its
> hind leg away from him to Port Largè. He sent its ribs
> from him to Dublin. . . . He turned his face northwards
> then, and went on thence to the summit of Sliab Breg,
> and he saw the peaks and knew the land of Cualnge,
> and a great agitation came over him at the sight of his
> own land and country, and he went his way towards
> it. In that place were women and youths and children
> lamenting the Brown Bull of Cualnge. They saw the
> Brown of Cualnge's forehead approaching them.
> "The forehead of a bull cometh towards us!" they
> shouted. . . . Then turned the Brown of Cualnge on
> the women and youths and children of the land of
> Cualnge, and with the greatness of his fury and rage
> he effected a great slaughter amongst them.[13]

This wasn't even the act of an aurochs, but of a domesticated bull.

Any animals this powerful were bound to excite the testes, so no-blemen liked to prove their nobleness by killing them. King Senacherib of Assyria is said to have hunted aurochs as early as the seventh century B.C., and the Romans went to great trouble to collect them for the arena. Charlemagne hunted them in A.D. 802, but by then the aurochs had already disappeared from all but Europe's darkest wilds. After the Middle Ages it was a short-lived, eastern curiosity, preserved for the pleasure of the Polish royals in the forest of Jaktorow, where it made its final stand.

There is a curious epilogue for the aurochs, three hundred years after their extinction. This happened, like many historical oddments, in Weimar Germany. Two brothers, Heinz Heck and Lutz Heck, at-tempted to breed the aurochs back to life by crossing "primitive" cattle breeds like the Spanish toros bravos with Scottish Highland, Hungar-ian Steppe, Frisian, and other strains. Heinz worked at the Hellabrunn Zoological Gardens in Munich; Lutz was director of the Berlin Zoo. In a Germany that was increasingly concerned with the science of genet-ics, this "back breeding" wouldn't have seemed too peculiar (the Nazis embraced Lutz's herd, applying racial politics even to cow husbandry). The Heck cattle, as the results are now known, never approximated the size of aurochs, but they did compose a few hot dinners for the broth-ers' starving countrymen in the aftermath of the war.

Heck cattle were a weird experiment, and nothing more. The truth is that there was no place for the aurochs in the modern world. It was too wild, too dangerous, and simply too big to fit into an age where all the land was stitched with fences. We needed our animals, like our serfs, to live quietly. That's why, for ten-thousand-odd years between the beginnings of animal husbandry and the death of the last aurochs, domestic cattle, not wild ones, have flourished, bred, and spread across the earth.

In the zoological tree, modern cows occupy a roost toward the upper foliage of the mammalian branch. Along with camels and peccaries, cows are members of the even-toed artiodactyl order, distinct for the symmetrical plane that passes between the third and fourth digits in their feet. Within this group, cattle belong to the bovid family, the hoofed beasts that wear frontal horns sheathed in keratin, a bonelike substance that accumulates throughout the life of the animal, as opposed to the pure-bone antlers annually shed by deer and their ilk. Goats, sheep, and gazelles are bovids.

Domestic cattle belong to the taxonomic subfamily bovinae, a class that embraces buffalo, bison, nyalas, elands, and bongos. The cow's genus, *Bos,* includes all oxen and yaks. *Bos taurus* is the Latinate for the European species of cattle, covering the breeds commonly known in the West, from Texas longhorns to Holsteins. Indian zebu (*Bos indicus*) are usually considered a separate species, but the classification is contested, and it's generally thought that both *Bos indicus* and *Bos taurus* descend from the aurochs, *Bos primigenius.* The main difference between *taurus* and *indicus,* apart from the Indian's shoulder hump and long, splayed ears, is the knack to survive in tropical climates. *Bos taurus* is a sluggard in the heat, and if dragged south is liable to stop giving milk before dying from some hothouse parasite. *Indicus* bows to no such frailties, and even boasts a resilience to ticks.[14]

Regardless of their difference, these two cousins share a common history, one that's part of the larger tale of how human beings gave up the spear and settled with the spade. It's the story of how we domesticated the natural world.

Before cattle or pigs or even goats came into our homes, dogs were our first allies. When the easy mammoths and "megafauna" of the Paleolithic died out, wolves and men learned that hunting in tandem meant a better chance of bringing down smaller, quicker game. As the wolves pattered around our camps, warmed their tails by our fires, and gnawed our leftover soup bones, we would have killed the aggressive ones, shooting them with arrows and skinning them for their fur. Over time, this culling would have favored wolves with more frolicsome personalities. They became more like pups, with short muzzles and a youthful taste for play.

Biologists Stephen J. Gould and Stephen Budiansky argue that this process, called neoteny, is common to many species.[15] Domestication favors animals that retain youthful traits like fearlessness, curiosity, and the ability to learn. Youthfulness also means less distinction between male and female—a reduction in what's called sexual dimorphism. Today (viewed from certain angles), modern domestic cows and bulls can appear practically identical. In contrast, an ancient aurochs cow was not only smaller and shorter horned than a bull, but wore a reddish-brown coat instead of a black one.[16] Cattle have about a fifteen-year generational cycle, so the process of reducing a brutish, unruly aurochs into a meek Frisian cow would have taken centuries.

Early dog domestication happened at a time when we still needed to catch our dinners, but subsequent domestications suited the new agricultural bent.[17] From about 10,000 B.C. to 8000 B.C. a group of opportunistic gazelle hunters called the Natufians started to build fixed settlements on the Anatolian plain in Turkey, a comfortable spot in the early world, and one happily overrun with foodstuffs. They harvested patches of wild cereals but didn't clear ground or plant seed, so they weren't technically agriculturists—at least not until after a thousand-year cold spell called the Younger Dryas had dried out the Middle East, shriveling the wild grains and forcing the Natufians to concoct a new way of feeding themselves. Over these frigid centuries, the shivering gatherers discovered that the foodstuffs they harvested began to change. The plants shed their defensive pathogens, swelled with edible seed and tissue, and became easier to reap and sow.[18]

This worked to both the advantage of these early Anatolian farmers as well as to the grains themselves. Biologist David Rindos says that a harvested plant is more likely to spread its seed than a plant left unpicked. Agriculture needed us, as much as we needed it. Wheat evolved to attract humans, just as flowers evolved to attract bees, and the result was a confluence of changing vegetation and human demand that sparked the dawn of agriculture around 7500 B.C. (at Jericho in the Levant, it may have been as early as 8000 B.C.). The first staples were emmer wheat, barley, rye, oats, and lentils, made lively on the plate by the addition of apples, onions, dates, figs, and garlic.

Cattle signed their symbiotic pact with humanity a little later. There are two broad theories as to how it happened, both of which likely hold part of the truth. The first is the "humongous pest" theory. With fields of grain budding outside their homes, the Neolithic farmers faced the problem of scavengers—not just birds and rodents, but also lumbering herbivores that would have eaten and trampled every fragile shoot of barley within scent. At first, the offended farmers probably roasted and boiled the trespassers, and we can imagine them ganging together to lie in wait to take revenge on a hoodlum aurochs. Eventually, the farmers realized that, instead of killing the vandals, they could corral them and eat them later.[19] Once penned, the most aggressive animals earned first place on the butcher's block, and over generations their rowdiest traits receded into genetic memory. The descendants were more pliant. This process would have taken centuries, but such is the pace of genetics.

The second theory of animal domestication is based on weather. Just like the Younger Dryas did a few millennia earlier, around sixty-four hundred years ago a second postglacial climatic shock parched the Middle East with a ruinous drought. Fields, newly seeded with the fruits of human ingenuity, withered, and people abandoned the settled, agricultural experiment, thinking the whole business a deathtrap.[20] While the rains had been kind and the fields moist, investing in wheat fields had made sense.[21] Now the hungry farmers would have looked back at the animals pasturing on the margins of the tilled land. They would have noticed that if a pasture turns brown or a valley is iced by a squall, a cow can walk to the next one. A lentil cannot.

So it's likely that the vagaries of climate first encouraged people to cultivate grain in the Younger Dryas, and then, when the weather turned bad again, it spurred them to hedge their bets by herding live-stock. Animals were a good way of "spreading their investments" in case of a collapse in the expected order of the universe. Shooing their herds before them, people chased the rains. But even cattle weren't impervious to drought. Cows need better feed and more water than do sheep or goats, and archaeological records tell us that there was a dietary shift, over time, from eating grain, to eating beef, to the last resort of eating mutton.

There may even be some memory of this upheaval in the Bible. Before the desiccation of the Younger Dryas, the Levant was a garden paradise. It was flush with wild fruits, overflowing vines, and plump game stooping by clear, abundant springs. When Eden disappeared in the wind, Adam learned to cultivate seeds, to rely on his skills instead of on God's bounty. But hard work couldn't fend off a second drought, and so Adam's descendants took to wandering with their flocks in an unending search for fodder. The Bible perhaps provides an analogy on this point, too. Jealous because the Lord preferred animal sacrifice to wheat, the farmer, Cain, killed the shepherd, Abel, and was doomed to exile and roaming.

The Book of Genesis makes another point on the subject of eating meat. After the Flood, God finally permitted the Hebrews to consume animal flesh. Livestock, and cows, became central to the diet of the Chosen People.

◆ Meat, Milk, Muscle, *and* Dung ◆

Neolithic farmers must have dreamed of beef. Otherwise they wouldn't have gone to the trouble of trying to corral animals as dangerous as wild cattle. In the early Neolithic, there were no plows in need of oxen, so they didn't need cows for labor. More important, people didn't drink milk. Primitive cattle weren't generous at the teat, and the Near Eastern peoples ten thousand years ago lacked the necessary stomach enzymes to digest milk in adulthood, as lactose tolerance is a relatively new development in human evolution. Even today, adult milk drinkers are mostly north-central Europeans descended from the Neolithic "Funnel Beaker" culture or East Africans descended from particular pastoralist tribes.[22]

Babies, on the other hand, have never lacked gusto for digesting milk and are not too picky about what sort of mammal provides it. Animal wet nurses arrived in the early years of domestication. The day that some thirsty child got the inkling to grab an idle udder was one of those unrecorded milestones in history, like striking fire out of a rock or punting in a hollow log.

Cows' milk changed us. Throughout our long walk out of hominid Africa, women of childbearing age and a modest coating of fat would have been continually pregnant or lactating. Only hunger, malnutrition, and ill health would have slowed the fertility rate, but with our domestication of the natural world, we obtained new sources of food. Cows' milk, which is high in protein and fat—two ingredients that are especially important for infant and maternal nutrition—allowed our species to leap wholeheartedly into perpetual rutting. Human fertility rebounded; women shortened their reproductive cycle and gave birth to more children. The effects on society would have been incalculable. Human beings, their numbers already swelling under a diet of grain, bred faster and better sustained their infants during the perilous years of infancy. Populations boomed. The wheels of civilization began to turn.

Gourds of ready milk were also an enticing foodstuff for adult humans, and over the Neolithic millennia, we bred adult lactose tolerance into several of our own gene pools. Either through desperate hunger or simple greed, we forced our stomachs to adapt, drowning our bellyaches in cream. Recent studies claim that early milk drinkers left ten times as many descendants as their abstemious siblings.[23] In the case of East Africans, the lactose mutation occurred as recently as three thousand years ago—an astounding instance of physical change in response to culture. We evolved because we wanted to drink cows' milk. Genetic selection worked simultaneously on our cows as they became domesticated, and on us. So the presence of cows, in the most direct manner imaginable, steered human evolution into a particular mutation.

We weren't, however, quite done with the cow. Drinking its mammary secretions and roasting its flesh was a good start, but human beings are opportunists. To a Neolithic cattle herder, living next to a half ton of animal muscle would eventually have raised the question: "How can I exploit this creature before I flay it, eat it, and carve its bones into utensils?"

Oxen are defeated things, more malleable than donkeys or camels. Even before the invention of the wheel, they would have been used to carry loads and thresh grain (Deuteronomy 25:4 mentions oxen treading grain).[24] Farmers had employed the simple hoe since the beginning of agriculture, and when the Bronze Age arrived, a technological leap in Mesopotamia yielded wheels and plows. Oxen were the muscle behind the machines. Spokes turned, furrows rose, and the earth produced ever broader, more bounteous fields under the trundling hooves of progress.

These fields needed to be fertilized, and, again, cattle took on the job. Civilization, as any cynic or student of agriculture will tell you, is built on dung. Without it, the Fertile Crescent wouldn't have been worth the name, because, after a few years of tillage, crops deplete the soil's natural levels of nitrogen. River flooding helps, but manure has always been fertility's dark agent. The shrewd farmers on the Euphrates were privy to the knowledge that the richest fields were the ones on which an animal had shat, and cattle are capable defecators—the manure from a modern dairy cow contains 0.7 percent nitrogen, adding up to eleven pounds of nitrogen per ton of fresh droppings. To a subsistence farmer with few resources save for his ox and prayers, this is gold and manna combined. In the developing world today, a plentiful dungheap can still mean the difference between a green field and starvation.

Cows needed people to tend them. Someone had to drive the herds, squirt the dugs, and cut the throats of these amazingly useful animals,

especially as cattle and human beings alike bred in denser, more intimate clumps around Near Eastern villages. Here is where the cowherd
enters history, first as a lowly attendant to the farmer, but, over time,
growing to cast a very long shadow. Herders constitute neither the
world's oldest profession nor indeed the second oldest. But they are the
most historically divisive.

As cattle herds crowded the corrals of Neolithic towns, a few ruined
crops would have made it evident that cows needed to live apart, to
graze somewhere far from the farmers' priceless stalks of wheat. Livestock needed pasture, and since the tilled land lay closest to the settlements, the boys and layabouts and dreamers who preferred watching
animals to picking shoots would have walked their charges out to the
pastures and into the wild. Over time, the mesh of tillage swelled, and
the herders led their beasts deeper into the unclaimed hinterland. And,
over time, the herders became a folk apart.

History is a sundered chain, a sequence of broken links between
peoples and ideas. None was more traumatic than the break between
farmers and herdsmen. It began innocently enough as a simple divide
of labor: one brother watched the herds while the other weeded the
fields. As the centuries passed, the herders learned to tell different stories, eat different foods, wear different clothes, and pray to different
gods. They lived under leather, as their ancestors did on the Mammoth
Steppe, and they became sharp-eyed and quick with arrows. They would
have felt no twinge of hesitation at taking a knife to a bleating calf.

They also began to speak with different words. Military historian
Robert O'Connell recounts this prehistoric divide between the agrari-
ans and the pastoralists—a fracture in human society that he thinks
only really healed in the past two hundred years, with the creep of industry. He tells us that the Neolithic pastoralists abandoned the coasts
and river basins to their homebound cousins, walking north or east
out of the memory of settled lands. This took time. For many generations the herders would have regularly come home to civilization, but
at some point around 6000 B.C., Neolithic society split between the
farmers and the herdsmen.[25]

Seen in this context, the story of Cain and Abel is a fable of this earliest of rivalries, and it's telling to note that Cain, the villain, was the farmer. A different version exists in the Sumerian myth of the goddess Inanna choosing between her suitors, Dumuzi the shepherd[26] and Enkimdu the farmer, a dispute that resulted in some of the most torrid poetry to survive from the ancient world, predating Solomon and Sheba's Song of Songs.[27]

> *My vulva, the horn*
> *The Boat of Heaven,*
> *Is full of eagerness like the young moon.*
> *My untilled land lies fallow.*
> *As for me, Inanna,*
> *Who will plow my vulva?*
> *Who will plow my high field?*
> *Who will plow my wet ground?*
> *As for me, the young woman,*
> *Who will plow my vulva?*
> *Who will station the ox there?* [28]

Dumuzi, evidently. The goddess picks the animal tender ("the wild bull") over the farmer as her bridegroom, an early victory for pastoralist manhood. (Interestingly, Dumuzi is an archetypal "Dying God" as well as a shepherd, and is identified with the annual blossoming of vegetation in the desert. He's also associated with the Bull of Heaven/ Taurus, which disappears for six weeks below the Sumerian horizon during the period of January through March—at the beginning of the Sumerian year.)

Cain and Abel were, of course, rivals of a different nature, vying for the favor of God himself. Cain's fratricide, the myth of the herdsman and the farmer at odds, endured longer than any other story in civilization, save that of the most ancient tale of all: of paradise lost.

―――――――――

◆ Pity *and* Fear ◆
Ernest Hemingway's Bullfights

Ernest Hemingway, who, when it came to things Spanish, was a cool disseminator of mistruths, made perhaps his sole foray into intentional humor with *Death in the Afternoon,* his study of the bullfight. Forgoing the crabbed severity that he cultivated in his fiction, Hemingway wrote about "tauromachia" with wit and an uncustomary panache. There's a very funny passage in which he asks his imaginary readers whether they enjoyed their first view of a bullfight (*corrida de toros,* literally "running of the bulls"). He imagines that they did not, with the exception of a weird old woman who considers the spectacle of bulls goring horses to be "sort of homey."[29]

Many of Hemingway's readers would have assumed that bullfighting is aberrant and cruel. They missed the point. Bullfighting isn't a sport "in the Anglo-Saxon sense of the word," meaning an equal contest with fair play and no ordained outcome. To think of it within the same context as football would render it not only gross, but immoral. Such an attitude, to Hemingway, is folly. He thought that morality could only be weighed by how something makes you feel. To him, the bullfight was moral because "I feel very fine while it is going on and have a feeling of life and death and mortality and immortality."[30]

This is a very good way to describe tragic art.

Art can be repellent. Art can offend. And the bullfight is undoubtedly capable of inciting nausea. But the *Oxford English Dictionary* defines art as "an application of skill according to aesthetic principles." Even the most disgusted witness to a bullfight must agree that the spectacle is as aesthetically principled as *Swan Lake.* What art cannot do is leave its audience unmoved.

That doesn't mean it can be explained. The Spanish acknowledge that there's mystery inherent in reenacting a semipagan slaughter. They have a proverb that says, "Not even the cows understand the bulls." Contradictions abound—the bulls are both lauded and tortured, subjected to knives and honest tears. No matter how hard Spaniards try to explain their relationship with the bulls—and there are university faculties devoted to the task—they always resort to airy maxims, shrugs, and poetry. To the language of faith. In the sixteenth century, a poet named Adolfo de Bonilla wrote:

> An earth-colored bull
> Boasts highly about
> Putting an end to our dusty weakness.
>
> He roars in the bullring,
> His strength leaving him,
> Facing the illustrious balcony
> Where the king is sitting.
>
> He fights many sad and bloody stages
> In the absence of a strong arm whom his fury
> could defeat.[31]

The poem is called "Romance of the Birth of Christ."

The typical bullfight, like many other tragedies, occurs in three acts. The opening act introduces the players when the bull erupts from his gate. For the first time in his life, the animal sees a man standing on foot instead of sitting on horseback or in a jeep. This alien figure is the matador, the hero bullfighter (torero) who will deliver the sword in the third act. He's distinct from the other toreros in his troupe (cuadrilla) by virtue of his expertise, his courage, and his outrageous suit, which looks like something Nureyev might have worn if he'd swapped the Ballet Russe for a Carnival float in Rio.

The bull initiates the spectacle by attempting to gore the matador. He fails, and the matador confounds him by twirling a broad, colorful dress cape. This is done to judge the bull's character—to see which horn he favors, whether he charges smoothly or in swerves, and whether he's drawn to a particular spot in the ring. Once the matador gets a sense of the animal, two mounted lancers (picadors) trot into the ring. Finally recognizing a target worthy of his horns, the bull happily charges the horses, which, unlike in Hemingway's day, are protected by padding. As the horse is pushed and lifted, the picadors impale the bull's neck, leaning into their weapons to bleed him. Steaming, the bull continues to buckle down and drive his head into the horse's ribs, ignoring his own deepening cuts. Without these wounds, he would be too frantic to allow the matador use of his more dramatic flourishes later on, but the spectacle is brutish, and is always the least loved part of the corrida, eliciting jeers from the spectators if the picadors press their lances too hard.

The second act is more florid. Three toreros called banderilleros sprint up to the bull and, like mosquitoes, jam barbed sticks in his back. They compete to deliver their barbs with the greatest flourish and the most ostentatious risk. Sometimes, when the banderilleros lose their nerve, they merely dart up to the bull's side and jab, but usually they twist and leap like salmon on a line. Blood spreads through the animal's coat, his raw back glistens, and his strength ebbs, readying him for the inevitable conclusion.

Now the matador enters the ring alone, armed with a sword and the light, red cape (muleta) of popular imagery. For the next fifteen minutes, the man leads the bull in a series of formalized passes, working as close to the horns as his skill and cojones permit. It ends when the matador positions the exhausted bull directly in front of him, its forelegs parted and shoulders exposed at just the perfect angle for a thrust. Then he slides his sword through the yielding tissue between the shoulder blades, arcing his own body past the bull's driving right horn. This is the moment of highest danger for the man, and, if performed well, it's the instant in which the sword enters the bull's aorta, killing it.

That's the elementary structure of the tragedy, but it's played out in infinite permutations. There are terrifying, twelve-volume encyclopedias that chart each twist of the muleta, every historical variance between the Ronda and the Seville schools of technique, the name for each gradation of a bull's horn, coat, and muzzle. The one fixed point is the tip of the matador's sword. Death is inexorable and fated, and it will have its victim. Pity and fear will be expunged.

◆ The Coconut Theory *of* Animal Husbandry ◆

Inside Pedro Trapote's farmhouse, along with lots of severed bulls' heads, groves of antlers, and a whole stuffed leopard, are some awesomely bad oil paintings. The one straddling the main stairwell is a nearly life-size portrait of the retired Andalusian bullfighter Curro Romero. Although he was a colossus of the bullring, as virile and steely as any man who's ever worn spangles, Romero lacks the morphology of a hero—he looks like a sort of wading bird. In the painting he stands naked save for a senatorial toga, his thin legs braced in a manly pose like a warrior consul or, more likely, a man about to commit something unlawful in a schoolyard. It's a breathtakingly unfortunate portrait, but a few feet away, next to the master bedroom, there's one that's even worse.

This is another nude, one in the style of high kitsch via El Greco and the supple Roman boy-god Antinous. It shows a curly-haired youth caught bullfighting, naked, in the moonlight. He's being led away by the civil guards (read Roman legionnaires), and as he descends from his private Calvary into the hammy grip of the policemen, his angular, sensuous face glows with the serenity of the martyr. His skin glows somewhat blue.

As silly as this painting is, it does catch a shade of the bullfighter's soul. There is no nobility in courting death. Any feckless schoolboy can do that. But there is beauty in mastering a force as potent as a bull's, in controlling it, and in paying homage to the bull's strength at the risk of one's own life. Or at least at the appearance of risk. A professional bullfighter ought never to feel a scratch. His command of the animal should be complete. The greatest bullfighter of all time was Pedro Romero of Ronda, called by Hemingway "the perfect male." He was the first torero to treat his work as an art instead of a mere show of bravura, and by the time he died at the age of eighty-five, he had killed more than six thousand bulls. His body didn't bear a single scar.

Bullfighting paintings aren't necessarily atrocious. The most famous example of good bullfighting art is "La Tauromaquia," a series of thirty-three etchings by Francisco de Goya. Goya was a champion misanthrope—which among Spanish artists is saying something—a bleak soul who saw the world riddled with toadstools. He had cause. Spain in the early nineteenth century was a bloody mire, overrun by war and destitution, and Goya vented his despair through black, even obscene paintings of cannibal titans, drooling princes, and braying peasants cracking one another's skulls with hard sticks. His bullfighting art, however, wasn't censure. It was journalism. The etchings evoke the vibrancy of nineteenth-century bullfighting—its costumes and acrobatics and wild swerves of fortune. The bulls are as fluid as the ones underground in Lascaux, but are infinitely less impressionistic. Goya had a correct eye for cow anatomy.

In "La Tauromaquia," Goya draws an island of nobility and grace in a sea of evils. So loving are his sketches that every year the elite of Spain—the descendants of the very aristocrats whom Goya caricatured with such inspired spleen—dress up in antique outfits for a festival of Goya-era bullfights. Even today, the event is one of the wildest media frenzies of the year, with social columnists crowding out the throngs of bullfighting critics. And these are indeed throngs. Among sports, bullfighting in Spain is second only in popularity to football. Except that it's not a sport.

"It's regulated by the Ministry of the Interior," says David Casas, a journalist who covers bulls for Madrid's Radio Union. That puts it in the same company as the Civil Guard and highway administration, as opposed to sports, which are overseen by the Ministry of Culture. Casas is thin and blue-jeaned and cultivates the hairy, sleepless dishevelment popular among Madrileños under forty. He looks like an unlikely champion for an activity as loaded with conservative, even nationalistic, associations as bullfighting. But then, it's a very modern business. Spanish bullfighting today generates 1.5 billion euros per year. About forty-five million spectators attend two-thousand-odd fights, supporting two hundred thousand jobs and fifteen hundred working bull farms.[32]

The history of the ring wasn't always so profitable. In the eighteenth and nineteenth centuries, most toreros entered the arena out of desperation. They were country boys, often Gypsies, who risked their lives for the price of a week's bread. Today's famous matadors can earn 180,000 euros per appearance. In the Spanish celebrity heavens, bullfighters shine brighter than actors and are on a par with aristocrats, whom they usually marry. The Duchess of Alba, a twisted stick of rarified DNA with more titles than the Queen of England, counts bullfighters among her relations.

Bullfighting has come full circle. Its modern form began with aristocratic knights training for crusades against the Moors. The wild bulls that ranged across Spain eight hundred years ago provided an excellent test of lancing, horsemanship, and mettle—the educational value of which didn't pass unnoticed to the Moors, who likewise hunted them. Indeed, the Moors are sometimes credited with starting the whole thing in the first place. Christian or Moor, what's certain is that bullfighting today is a child of the Middle Ages.

But then, so was the Black Death. Why should modern secular Europeans—sensible social democrats who buy kitchen sets at IKEA and avoid spiritualism like they would a lurching, talkative drunk—pay to watch a ceremonial bloodletting?

"Suffering exists," says Casas. "Walt Disney got it wrong."

One of the authors recalls going to his first corrida, fought by a rising young fighter called El Fundi. He fully expected to be repelled by the experience, like one of Hemingway's despised dilettantes who always made a "well-fed, . . . beach-tanned, flannelled, Panama-hatted, sport-shod exit" after the first kill.

He did not. What he saw was a man kneeling in the blazing sand, his arms spread as if he were trying to embrace the sun. Then, an animal force bore down upon him like a wave, bent on breaking him to pieces. Up he sprang, and he danced the bull through a flight of whirls and veronicas, shaping the bull's power with a touch and flash of the cape, proving that he was alive and that there was still something glorious left to do in a life built of gas bills, shopping carts, and advertisements.

This is bullfighting's appeal. It's an act that, when done well, can remind the audience that life is—still—sublime.

After his fashion, Trapote agrees. "It's not rational," he says. "In the twenty-first century, what is a guy doing dressed like a woman in pink tights and a very ugly hat, wearing a suit that weighs more than his mother? It's not rational! The world of the bull is not rational!"

Nor are the economics, particularly. Regardless of the industry's billions of euros in revenue, perhaps only 10 percent of all ranchers like Trapote actually make money on their stock. It costs more than 3,500 euros to raise a toro bravo to full age, but only about 20 percent of a given year's bulls ever fetch the high prices paid by prestigious arenas like Madrid or Seville. The rest—through poor temperament or physical imperfections—are sold cheaply to lesser venues, village fairs, or even straight to the butcher's block. For Trapote, these animals lose money.

"I could raise a pig for one year and sell it for 600 euros," he scoffs. Instead, he raises bulls for two, three, or four years. He's lucky to get a thousand for most of them.

Trapote explains his business philosophy with the story of the coconut.

"A man went up a palm tree and got a coconut. He opened the coconut, drank the milk, and ate the meat. Suddenly, an American showed up. You know, Americans are more pragmatic, and he says, 'Why don't you go up and get the coconut, and sell it to me?'

" 'What for?' asks the man.

" 'With the money you can hire five people to pick coconuts, and then you build a bar, a chiringuito, on the beach.'

" 'What for?'

" 'When you've built the chiringuito, you build a factory to put the coconut milk in a tin can. Then you sell it to the city.'

" 'But what for?'

" 'Then, when you have three hundred people working for you, you sell the coconut milk worldwide.'

" 'What for?'

" 'Well, to make money.'

" 'But why do you want to make money?'

" 'So you can come here and enjoy life.'

"The man considers this and replies, 'But what do you think I'm already doing?' "

◆ The Reddest Meat *of* All ◆

Two blocks from the arabesque bullring of Las Ventas in Madrid stands a restaurant that marks the final resting place of countless slaughtered bulls. Specializing in roast kid and *carne de lidia* ("meat of the bull-fight"), Casa Toribio's dining room is a formal, muted pink, and the walls are festooned with faux-impressionist bull art. The best table is even overlooked by a clubby piece of pornography: a cheesecake blonde, naked but for lace garters and a torero's open jacket, toying with a horned bull. During corrida season, it takes two weeks to book a lunch. Otherwise, the restaurant is populated by a clique of dapper cardplayers who strain against their tailored waistbands, drink colored liquors, and smoke pipes.

Above them, cross-armed and genial, stands the owner of the place, Toribio Anta Anta. He looks like Bill Clinton's Castilian cousin, down to the twinkling squint and cigar. And he's built a career on bull meat.

"The flesh is very fibrous and very strong," explains Toribio. Toros bravos that never saw the inside of an arena, like the females, are bargains at a mere 150 euros per carcass. "They don't sell much of it here. Most of the meat goes to Russia, but the South Americans and the Chinese markets buy it, too." Toribio isn't concerned with thrift. His dishes have all died in combat in the arena, which infuses them with a cachet worth 25 euros for a plate of stew. His restaurant has cornered

Las Ventas's supply of bull tail, the most prized cut from a fighting animal, and which is sometimes awarded to the matador for an exceptional performance in the arena. Usually, though, it goes into Toribio's refrigerator.

He shows off a vacuum-sealed package of what appears to be red eels. They're actually three kilos of tail cut from bulls that died in the arena at Valladolid two months ago.

Once a bull receives its estocada—its killing blow—the carcass is dragged, to the accompaniment of trumpets, across the sand by a team of mules. Out of sight, the body is hauled to a refrigeration truck, which whisks it from the eighteenth-century atmosphere of the bull-ring and into a modern inspection facility off one of the six-lane highways spinning out of Madrid. After a government inspector deems it edible, a butcher removes what's left of the tenderloin (a cut frequently ruined by sword wounds and bandilleras), slices off the steaks, and, most important, snips off the tail. It's a long cylinder of spindled bone, sheathed in gristle and dark filaments. This is then aged for at least ten days. Toribio cooks his bull's tail stew according to the following Andalusian recipe.

≈⌀≈

CULINARY INTERLUDE

Bull's Tail Stew

Chop two pounds of meat into discs about two inches thick, which you soak in coarse red wine (Sangre de Toro is best) for twelve hours. When the flesh is tender, brown it in olive oil with diced onions, tomatoes, carrots, and mushrooms. Transfer the meat and vegetables to a large stewpot, and simmer in white wine. Cook for three hours, reducing the vegetables to a salty, maroon gravy. Serve on a bed of diced potatoes.

The meat is fatty and black, and it is so thickly veined with gelatin that the texture approximates pudding. Like stews made from the bull's lesser cousin, the ox, this dish takes its flavor from the bone. The filaments, which flake off the starfish-shaped vertebrae at the approach of a fork, have almost blended with the marrow, giving the flesh a taste of sweetmeats without the iron tang. This strength complements the dense, concentrated sauce—a weaker meat would be overwhelmed by the paste of onions and carrots. It's a powerful, robust stew.

Although tail is the most prestigious dish, Toribio serves other bull meat in season, like grilled tenderloin in red wine. Fighting bull steaks demand a deft hand with the fire. The meat is lean, lacking the marbling of beef, and is nearly purple in color. This intensity of red is partly due to the animal's muscularity, but also because it dies in a state of furious stress, flushing the tissue with lactic acid. Since it lacks an insulating spiderweb of fat, bull steak quickly overcooks, so it's best served rare. Grilled with pepper and salt, it has a concentrated flavor, like consommé, but without the greasier texture of richer cuts (in the United States, the closest substitute is bison).

Since bull is grass-fed and lean, it's one of the healthiest meats available. It's also ecologically sound and toros bravos are raised without use of chemical fertilizers, hormone injections, or genetically modified food. The land they inhabit is virginal, looking no different than it did in the reign of Philip II. It practically thrums with partridges. Of the three hundred thousand hectares of Spanish farmland devoted to toros bravos, all are untouched by pesticides, while the bulls never sniff a chemical or an unsound bite of feed. During the mad cow scare of 2000–2001, not a single toro bravo contracted the disease.

◆ Delamere's Cattle ◆

Ten miles from the balloons and elephants of the Masai Mara National Reserve, the savanna dips into a wooded prairie where cows take shade by a brackish stream. In the middle of the road, they huddle in their dusty hundreds—red or speckled, black or chestnut, but all of them low-slung and slender, with their zebu humps bunched like mushrooms at the shoulder blades. Jerry, our Masai driver, slowed and rolled down his window as two eight-year-old boys, barefoot in red cloaks, hurried to look inside our car and ask for money. They carried heavy iron spears. For the lions.

"It used to be that warriors would go out to the Mara and hunt the lion, to become brave and strong," said Jerry, who intimated that this was less a rite of manhood than a reasonable workout regimen. The Masai don't revel in metaphors about their warriors being as fierce as lions or as strong as bulls. Rather, they compare them to fire.

As we drove up the Narok road, we rattled through a neat mesh of wheat and cornfields framed by acacias whose blooms trailed like green wisps of smoke. There were cattle trundling in the dust at the roadside, sometimes poked along by boys even younger than our two callow spearmen. Jerry was talking about a story we had heard from the elders back in the village called Endikirt Osenyai. Leaning into their walking sticks, the old men had recounted a story from their past: the last great Masai cattle raid, an attack on the Kalinjen tribe that occurred during the 1960s. With no more fluster than if they had been remarking on the rain, these gray-headed elders spoke of killing "very many" people and chasing the survivors for fifty kilometers "before the government intervened."

Tribal violence is a common misery in Kenya, but usually it's over politics. These Masai had killed for cattle.

Jerry pointed at a hut nearly buried in a green swell of pasture. "That's where the raid took place," he said. It took little effort to imagine the last Masai battlefield there, the squads of trotting red cloaks and iron spears glinting in the yellow afternoon. And everywhere cattle, always cattle. That's the only reason the Masai ever fought.

"A Masai would die to take a cow," said Jerry. "He would give his life."

We stopped at the Member's Club in Narok for beer and Red Bull. It's a leafy campsite fronted by a jumble of shapeless whitewash and planking. There's a car-cleaning service and a pub. A man was throttling a chicken in an unlit doorway, and the waitress waved at Jerry from behind the bar's protective iron lattice. Jerry knew everyone, as usual.

The conversation drifted along, buoyed by the hot summer breeze, to less famous cattle raids and the legacies of English invaders.

"I have eaten Delamere's cattle," said Jerry. This was surprising. Lord Delamere was the colonial leader whose descendants still own one of Kenya's largest cattle operations, a forty-thousand-hectare holdover from the age of white gloves and whites-only whiskey bars. Its original lease, like that of other big, British-owned ranches in the Laikipia region, expired in 2004, and the Masai called for immediate eviction, threatening to take their case to the International Court of Justice in the Hague. Tempers are still raw. There have been killings, two of which involve the Delamere heir Tom Cholmondley, sparking a bonfire of televised rage. Since Delamere's cattle are stout Jersey milkers, unique among Kenya's millions of flat-teated zebus, it was odd that Jerry had eaten them.

"I was sixteen years old," said Jerry. "I wanted to experience the jungle life." It was 1976, he told us, long after the great raiding days of the Masai. He had walked for two days into the bush to join eight other boys and sixty-three warriors in a thieving party. They rustled about a hundred head.

"I stayed behind as a guard with the other boys while the warriors drove the animals off. We lived in a cave, eating meat every day. We boiled soup with herbs. Wild-making herbs, so your blood opens up and you no longer feel pain." For three months, Jerry lived the warrior life. He wrestled, ate skewered beef, and drank a broth of seketit seeds, olkiloriti bark, and olkitonusua root—the Masai equivalent of steroids.

"Those herbs are bad news. You become a bully. Fierce." The habitual smile, like a crescent moon, split his face. "You're wrestling someone, a friend, and thinking, 'I should be killing you!' "

Jerry and his companions were thieves, not proper Masai raiders. A generation before this, raids were still a formal undertaking, acts of robbery and murder constrained by ritual. The attack always began with the expectant warriors claiming a pair of cows from every house in their own village—a sort of military tax. Since they never planned for long campaigns, and since no one troubled with baggage, these animals were eaten on the spot, a process that itself could take months (King Solomon, who once cooked twenty-two thousand oxen for a dinner, would have made a good Masai). While fires guttered under the smoking brisket, the would-be raiders practiced wrestling, club fighting, and spear throwing, turning feral on a diet of meat and Jerry's frenzied herbs. Scouts ran out to the enemy villages, but not for reconnaissance. The intention was swagger and threat. "Surrender every cow, steer, and heifer," the scouts would say, "or the Masai will kill you all."

If the enemy chose to fight, the raiders finished chewing the gristle and lapping the blood, and, on the morning of departure, each man would take a walk alone in the forest, carrying the stick on which he had roasted his food. This he pushed into the ground to thank God for the meat. He prayed:

"My God, I have come out. Me, a poor man. Me, whose clothes hang loose. It is only you who can tighten my clothes. My spear will remain intact because you have decided it. My white morning, given by God who supersedes all nations, let me reach old age when my buttocks will have shrunken!"

The warrior also prayed for his lazy comrade, still lying asleep after the feast:

"It is not his fault! He involved himself with alcohol and girls! God, prevent me from becoming a womanizer."

After being blessed with consecrated milk, the men jogged into the brush, to war.

The greatest cattle raid of all time happened about 150 years ago, when the Ildamat clan attacked another Masai clan, the Isiria. The Ildamat are scanty today, but then they once were powerful enough to circumcise nine thousand boys before the battle. They crushed the Isiria and launched a hundred raids against all the other seventeen clans. Although the fighting lasted more than a month, the Masai don't celebrate any individual decapitations or heroic butcheries. But they still sing songs about the size and beauty of the cows that the warriors brought home.

Shortly after this Great Raid, the Ildamat met their nemesis in a flush of smallpox. Thousands died, and the clans, still tottering from the Great Raid, were conquered by their irksome northern cousins, the Laikipiaks. The Masai, keen ironists all, still nod their heads and sigh over the disaster.

At the end of his warrior summer of 1976, Jerry turned his back on the robbers' cave and took the long walk out of the Iron Age. He left his home and parents and moved into the twentieth century. There was a future to consider, and no one ever passed a civil service exam by squatting in a cave over rustled bones. University men don't wrestle in the ash of cookfires. Veterinarians don't fight with clubs. But even thirty years later, when the dumb squawk of traffic and the insolence of fools leave him feeling low or sour, Jerry Ole Kina sometimes walks into the starry woods to pluck the bitter herbs. He brews his potion on a stovetop, and he imbibes the fury of youth. Just to remember.

2

THE FOOD OF THE GODS

The Origin of Religion:
8000 B.C.–400 B.C.

◆ Bull Gods *on* Hadrian's Wall ◆

In A.D. 122, Emperor Hadrian paid an official call on the Roman province of Britain. No emperor had visited the island since Claudius added it to the empire several generations earlier, but Hadrian had good reason to risk the channel crossing from Germany. His legions had just quashed a British revolt—one of many that had bloodied the province since its annexation—and he wanted to put a permanent end to the troubles. So he decided to fix the northern border of the empire at the thin neck of the island. To the south, there would be a land of law, industry, and commerce. To the north, there would be hooting Picts.

For the next six years, Roman soldiers hauled turf, mortar, and limestone through the boggy grass of the Tyne Valley and across the Great Whin Sill, a giant escarpment of basaltic rock that cuts through the sod of Northumberland, just south of Scotland. The resulting wall spanned seventy-three miles between the Solway Firth and the Tyne estuary—a fortification too long to be defensible, but strong enough to modulate the ebb and flow of people and contraband. "Mile castles" and turrets stood at measured intervals. Sixteen fortresses housed the garrisons, and they brought with them drainage, marketplaces, plumbing, and the Romans' storied bathhouses. They also brought permanence. The legionnaires who came to live on the wall were there for good.

To a shivering clerk from Arles or a blue-fingered trumpeter from Cadiz, life along the wall must have been alien and sunless. The steam baths would have helped, and the exiles must have learned to stomach the local Celtic beer, to which the garrisons became addicted.[1] In Alan K. Bowman's collection of the surviving correspondence from the wall, we glimpse a provincial backwater, more dull than truly wretched, but nonetheless a lonely last resting place at the end of the earth.

To combat the ennui, some of the soldiers took to prayer. In Carrawburgh (ancient Brocolitia), at the northernmost point of the wall, you can still walk through the foundations of a small rectangular temple dedicated to a very unusual god.

The temple is small, no more than a few dozen steps lengthwise across a sward on which roosts a little weathered altar. As an archaeological site, it's modest, even paltry. The god of the temple wasn't even British. He came from the East, and his initiates believed in personal salvation through the blood of a sacred victim. They felt an intimacy with their deity, thinking he took the time to listen to individual prayers. His worship culminated in a symbolic meal, eaten in communion, in which the initiates broke bread and drank wine to reenact a scene from their god's mythology. The religion promised a golden afterlife, so it was especially appealing to slaves, freedmen, and the plain soldiery—to the humble and the meek.

The god's name was Mithras, and his followers, who were always men, raised his shanty temples in slums and border towns throughout the empire. It's estimated that at the peak of Mithras's popularity in the

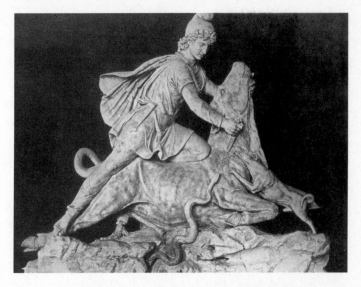

A STATUE OF THE GOD MITHRAS SLAYING A SACRED
BULL. *Credit: Original publication from the Vatican
Museum Collection. Photo by Hulton Archive/Getty
Images.*

second and third centuries, seven hundred temples crouched, sequestered among the thrumming brick alleys of Rome and its port city,
Ostia. Multiply this by vastness of the Roman Empire, and Mithras's
adherents must have been very numerous indeed.[2]

Mithras was a bull slayer, a cattle thief, and a sun god. In art, we
usually see him as a young man dressed in Persian garb, wrestling a
great bull while stabbing a dagger into its side. As the bull dies, an ear
of wheat sprouts from where its tail should be, while watching the
tussle is a motley gang of astrological figures: a dog, a scorpion, a raven,
the sun and the moon. Behind the scene, a cave mouth yawns open, a
passage into a deeper world.

Mithras's temples were modeled on this cave and were very different from those of the popular state gods like Apollo or Jupiter whose
temples boasted biologically correct marbles, fluted columns, and se-
renely ordered beauty. His adherents needed no such frivolities—just
stone hunkered against the black, northern wind; deliberately graceless

like the natural sanctums of the inner earth. Caves, like labyrinths, are purely interiors. They have no outward character. What's important is inside. When entering the chambers, Mithras's worshippers may have remembered Theseus, who transformed from a boy into a hero by creeping underground and, alone in the cold shadows, facing the Minotaur. The painters of the Lescaux bulls, too, made a physical descent and underwent their artistic contortions in the dark.

What happened inside Mithras's temples was a reenactment of a mythological dinner. Mithras's art repeatedly shows a sacred picnic, often depicted on the reverse of the bull-sacrifice relief. Using the slain animal's skin as a blanket, the god shared a feast with Sol, the sun, before the pair ascended together into the heavens. Mithraic initiates gathered in their "caves" to eat, reclining on platforms that faced each other across a central aisle. They broke bread and drank wine and dressed in pieces of costume denoting their rank in the cult—"Lion" or "Persian" or "Father." When they sacrificed a bull—a treat, since Pliny the Elder tells us that bulls are "the most extravagant way of appeasing the gods"[3]— they roasted the beef as a sacred barbecue. More regularly, they would have eaten cheaper dishes like ground meat and sausage.

☜☞

CULINARY INTERLUDE

A Mithraic Dinner with Meatballs

The Romans were never a beef people. They loved paler meats: fowl, fish, and pork. The culinary author Apicius writes, in his catalog of meats:

> *Entrees of peacock occupy the first rank, provided they*
> *be dressed in such a manner that the hard and tough*
> *parts be tender. The second place in the estimation*
> *of Gourmets have dishes made of rabbit. Third spiny*
> *lobster. Fourth comes chicken and fifth young pig.*[4]

A Mithraic dinner menu, being humble, may have sometimes included Apicius's common meatballs: isicia omentata.

Although Apicius would have preferred ground pork, ground beef works well for this dish. Combine one pound beef with two table-spoons bread crumbs (Apicius uses "the hearts of winter wheat"), a tablespoon of crushed pine nuts, pepper and salt, and a dash of red wine. Apicius also adds myrtle berries, but these can be substituted by (somewhat) more accessible juniper berries, or green peppercorns. A tablespoon will do.

Form the mixture into small patties and fry in an oiled skillet on a medium heat. When cooked, remove the meatballs and add ½ cup of red wine and ½ cup beef stock to the skillet. Add 2 tablespoons fresh thyme, a few peppercorns, and boil for several minutes, until reduced to a suitable gravy. Pour over the meatballs. For added authenticity, serve with a jolt of bottled Vietnamese fish sauce, the closest relative to the ubiquitous Roman seasoning called garum.

Eighty miles to the southeast of the ruins of Mithras's temple, in the great legionary city of York, another foreign god celebrated a different form of communion, and does so to this day. This religion has proved more tenacious than Mithraism. Instead of a ruin in a sheep meadow, York boasts a Minster, a limestone splendor into which centuries of artistic energy have been channeled into stained-glass, sixty-meter towers, a forest of High Medieval sculpture, and the largest Gothic vaults in northern Europe. But as a lone, surviving Roman column at-tests, mounted just outside the Minster, the ground was once pagan. It was the site for the legionary principia, the city's military headquar-ters, where the army's holy eagle standards were housed, oiled, and venerated before being hoisted off to war. And it was on this spot, on July 25, 306, that Christianity defeated every other religion for domi-nance in the Roman world.

Emperor Constantius, who had spent the year campaigning against the intractable savages to the north of the wall, returned to York, where he died. Egged on by one Crocus, a wily German king in Roman service, the soldiers assembled before the principia and shouted their allegiance to his son, Constantine, demanding that he take up the imperial purple. He agreed, and led them south, to civil war. The rest of his tale—his vision before the Battle of Malvern Bridge in which (the Christian) God told him, "By this sign conquer!", how he painted crosses on his men's shields, his victory, his consolidation of power, and his proclamation of Christianity as the state religion of the empire—is the stuff of hagiography.

Among York Minster's florid bouquets of stained glass (the most famous, the Rose Window, isn't even religious, and shows the union of the Houses of Lancaster and York), there's a humdrum image of Saint Luke the Evangelist. It's found hidden amid a cacophony of medieval art in the thirteenth-century "chapter house," a large circular meeting hall just off the main body of the Minster. The image is unremarkable except for one element. At the beginning of the Book of Ezekiel, the prophet sees a vision of four winged creatures hurtling out of the storm clouds, monstrous heralds of the coming of Christ. Each has four faces, which tradition holds are representative of the four evangelists, the four books of the Gospel. Matthew's face is a man's. Mark's is a lion's. John's is an eagle's. And Saint Luke, frozen for centuries in York's ecclesiastic windowpanes, is forever tied to the symbol of the bull.

Mithras disappeared with the Romans, but the image of the sacred bull preceded him by many millennia and lasted long after his cult gave way to Christ. Bulls have been the center of cult since cult began. It was the bull that ignited the first sparks of religion, long ago in the unrecorded night of history.

◆   First Rites   ◆

About ten thousand years ago, a roving group of hunters decided to linger on a ridge above a marshy basin in what would one day become central Turkey. Now called Çatalhöyük, the ridge stood above a river flowing through a plain tufted with sedge and steppe grass. Seasonal ponds drew flocks of nesting waterfowl, and wild cattle and gazelle would stoop to drink among the bulrushes, bending graceful necks for hunters' arrows. On higher ground grew hackberry, pistachio, oak, and almond. There were fish, and eggs, and plants for fuel and thatching. The hunters stayed.

They didn't leave for fourteen hundred years, during which time they had changed from living as hunters and gatherers to being fully sedentary, farming people. They altered the landscape, too, by cutting forests and sowing fields. Their settlement grew to house as many as eight thousand souls, making Çatalhöyük one of the world's first urban centers. But it was a different sort of town than the walled fortress of Jericho, built far away to the south in the Levant. Çatalhöyük was a cluster of small, rectangular dwellings separated by middens. The houses were bunched so closely together that their roofs formed the streets and public areas of the town.

We can imagine the Çatalhöyükers hopping between rooftops, talking, playing, and whiling away the daylight hours in the sun, before climbing down ceiling ladders into their homes, which were smoky, dark, and somewhat eerie. The Çatalhöyükers buried their dead within the floors of their homes. Generations lived together, with the living sleeping above the bones of their ancestors.

Çatalhöyük is an archaeologist's plum. It yielded troves of information on Neolithic agriculture and the origins of sedentary culture, but it's as a source of early symbols that the site is unmatched. The most celebrated of its treasures are clay figurines—large numbers of them unearthed in spots as diffuse as grain bins and refuse pits. Many of these figurines depicted the sort of stylized, corpulent female body that's now familiar to readers of National Geographic: anonymous heads, globular torsos, and zeppelin breasts. Other nearby sites yielded similar figures, and they've long been thought of as evidence of a Neolithic fertility cult—the mother of Cybele, Aphrodite, and Venus—the Mother Goddess herself.[5]

Apart from tinkering in sculpture, the Çatalhöyükers had a liking for murals of vultures, leopards, and especially of bulls. One famous example depicts a colossal, red-coated bull being hunted by Lilliputian human figures, mere insects before the heaving bulk of their prey. Inside the dwellings, bulls often took more concrete form—horns and skulls were frequently embedded in the plaster, sometimes on the walls, but also in seemingly awkward spots on the floor or, even less comfortably, in the platforms that served as furniture. More so than the Mother Goddess dolls, bulls were part of home decor.

The astonishing prevalence of bull imagery in Çatalhöyük has fueled daring flights of scholarly conjecture, all vying with each other in trying to explain why people here lived as they did. The important point to remember is that, out of everything in the infinite realm of human experience and the natural world, the Çatalhöyükers liked to paint bulls and sculpt naked women. As we've seen in the Paleolithic caves, a lively interest in breasts and ungulates is apparently common to the human condition. But in Çatalhöyük, we can first see where fascination turns into cult.

It's impossible to pin down the moment when nature yielded gods out of a sunrise or demons from a wisp of fire, but organized cult and sedentism—the decision by human beings to live in a single place year-round—are twinned. One inflamed the other, like two burning sticks held together. So while it's easy to assume that Neolithic people gave up chasing herds of game simply because they realized they could eat better if they sat on a lush bed of mollusks, or a fishing ground, or a patch of wild wheat, the latest scholarship suggests that the truth is, as always, not so simple. Our ancestors had more on their minds than the stuff in their bellies.

In *The Goddess and the Bull,* Michael Balter, the biographer of the Çatalhöyük dig, writes that the site was ill suited for growing most of the domesticated grains that its inhabitants liked to eat.[6] Even more strangely, the town was seven miles distant from the nearest good source of oak and juniper, the dominant forms of timber. Why, then, would thousands of Neolithic farmers and builders decide to spend their lives there? Ian Hodder, a leader of the Çatalhöyük excavations, believes that the Çatalhöyükers settled on the spot because the soil nearby was rich with marl and alluvial clay—the mud from which plaster is made. You can't sculpt goddess figures and paint bull murals without plaster. The Çatalhöyükers, says Hodder, might have staked their claim less on account of easy access to water, food, or shelter but for plaster, for artists' materials. This leads, naturally, to the intriguing idea that human beings are more than just talking, warring, politicking, materialist primates. We are the doodling animal. And what we chose to doodle is very telling.

Despite a vegetable emphasis in their menu, Çatalhöyükers didn't sketch sheaves of wheat or landscapes with farmers plucking greenstuffs on the plains. Neolithic artists, like their Paleolithic predecessors, painted hunters chasing bulls. Troves of wild cattle bones have been discovered on the site, suggesting that the bull hunt, and then the subsequent feast of roast meat, was the peak of Çatalhöyük's social calendar and would have probably marked special occasions like a birth, or the construction of a new house. Whereas today we'll take a snapshot of our daughter's graduation dinner, a Çatalhöyüker would have plastered the main course's skull into the living room wall. It would have been a grand memento, like a framed diploma or a family portrait. But the horns were also immortalized dinner scraps. They reminded visitors that the household had once feasted its neighbors and was therefore deserving of respect.

In addition to making a banquet, Hodder believes that cattle were somehow connected to ancestor veneration. Anthropologist Linda Donley-Reid examined the Çatalhöyük artworks through the prism of psychoanalysis and concluded that cattle hunting may have been a male initiation rite, binding fathers to sons and men to the domestic community.[7] Cattle, whether as food, ritual object, or painter's muse, were on people's minds.

Why cattle, and not other useful animals? Goats and sheep, as we have seen, were domesticated earlier and would have been a common sight on the Konya plain. They're just as edible as cows, are much more

sociable, and they, too, sport flowing udders. Horses are just as mag-
nificent as bulls. Pigs are just as ferocious. It's true that poultry lack
mammalian charm, but it still seems arbitrary that cattle, out of all the
possible meat and dairy beasts, should be the ones to inflame the Neolithic spirit.

It's tempting to think that we worship that which we most fear, and
also what we most desire. A wild bull is a fearsome danger and a
prize—its hunter could be broken to pieces, but he may also have his
ton of flesh. Unlike dogs, sheep, and goats, the only specimens of cattle
known to Çatalhöyük were untamed. They belonged to the outside
world, to the wild earth, and hence to the unlit realm beyond the fire-
light. In *The Domestication of Europe,* Ian Hodder calls this realm the
agrios, the savage, which existed in Neolithic minds as the opposite of
the *domus,* the house and its civilizing rituals, its bits of cloth and pot-
tery, its blood ties. By dividing his worldview into these conceptual
opposites, our early ancestors laid the psychological foundations to
tame the world. Taming the bull, as we have seen, was more of a matter
of will than muscle.

A Neolithic hunter venturing into the *agrios* to stalk a gigantic,
powerful animal performed more than just a dietary act. The influential French historian Jacques Cauvin, in *The Birth of the Gods and the
Origins of Agriculture,* wrote that in prehistoric societies, "the image of
the wild bull signifies brute force, instinctive and violent, is spontane-
ous in us and is without doubt universal."[8] No hunter would have approached the prospect of a bull hunt without feeling some sense of
gravity. Fear had to weigh in the balance with a hunger for meat and
for social esteem.

Çatalhöyük is an exception, an early flowering of urban life that
withered from memory until *Archaeology* magazine resurrected it in a
full-color photo spread. Large populations didn't settle into city life
until much later. Cattle, however, did not disappear from the minds of
ancient Mediterranean peoples. They continued to exist as something
much more significant than four-legged banquets. A story from the

Mediterranean's greatest poet illustrates how cattle were food, certainly. But they were also touched by the divine.

◆ Early Myths *and* Legends ◆
The Cattle *of the* Sun *and the* Bull *of* Heaven

In Book XII of *The Odyssey,* Homer recounts how Odysseus's loyal sailors, after having weathered war, witches, whirlpools, and even the gates of Hades itself, finally succumb to a foreordained plot device. Having just seen six of their number eaten alive by the monster Scylla, the distraught crew lands on the "Thrinacian island," a land that later audiences probably recognized as Sicily. There, they see seven herds of cattle, flanked by seven herds of sheep. Odysseus, warned by the ghost of the prophet Teiresias, knows that these animals are not marked for mortal stomachs.

"Let us mind, therefore, and not touch the cattle," he tells his men. "Or we shall suffer for it; for these cattle and sheep belong to the mighty sun, who sees and gives ear to everything."

The sailors are not idiots. They do as they're told. Or they do for one long month while a southerly wind locks them in harbor. Their wine and grain run out, and the hungry men are reduced to snaring seabirds on the rocks. Finally, a clever fellow named Eurylochus presents an obvious argument: Why not sacrifice the cattle to the gods?

Sacrifice, to the Greeks, had a sly consequence. Celestial gods, they reasoned, best liked the smoke from burnt vitals (earthly, chthonic gods preferred their food buried). Olympians, even decorous Athena, took immense pleasure in snuffing at the oily residue of spleens. This was the fault of the titan Prometheus, who had long ago tricked Zeus into accepting the bones of sacrifices while people were left to enjoy the meat and the fat. This didn't mean that the Greeks didn't burn their sacrifices in a spirit of sincere piety. They did. But every offering meant a splendid dinner for the worshippers.

Eurylochus, therefore, tried to persuade his companions to sacrifice the Cattle of the Sun. The offering of burnt innards would presumably assuage the gods' anger, and then the sailors, happily fed, could always promise to build a big, shiny temple in thanks for the meat, once they arrived safely home. Besides, what could the gods do to punish them that would be worse than slow starvation? Better to risk the thunderbolts. The sailors, succumbing to their bellies, agreed. Homer tells us what happened:

> Now the cattle, so fair and goodly, were feeding not
> far from the ship; the men therefore drove in the best
> of them, and they all stood round them saying their
> prayers, and using young oak-shoots instead of barley-
> meal, for there was no barley left. When they had
> done praying they killed the cows and dressed their
> carcasses; they cut out the thigh bones, wrapped them
> round in two layers of fat, and set some pieces of raw
> meat on top of them. They had no wine with which
> to make drink-offerings over the sacrifice while it was
> cooking, so they kept pouring on a little water from
> time to time while the inward meats were being grilled;
> then, when the thigh bones were burned and they had
> tasted the inward meats, they cut the rest up small and
> put the pieces upon the spits.[9]

There are more refined dishes than beef thighs grilled in lard and basted with water. But to a starving man, watching his meal char on a guttering fire, the aroma must have been maddening. Homer says that when the Sun found his herd gobbled by mortals, he took his grievance to Zeus, threatening to hide his light in the underworld and cast the earth into withering darkness unless the sailors were punished. As was usual in mythical Greece, the outcome was both predicted and bloody. The sailors got the favorable wind for which they'd prayed, but they had barely set sail before Zeus blasted their ship into smithereens. Everyone except for Odysseus drowned in the wine-dark sea.

The lesson in Homer's story isn't just the cliché of "leave the gods well enough alone." Despite the ivory, moonlike crescents of their horns, cattle have a purity of strength, like fire. Like the sun. And to the ancient solar deities—be he Helios, Hyperion, Ra, or Mithras—cows were sacred. The cows that the sailors ate in desperation were no mere beast, but the symbolic embodiment of the sun itself. No wonder he got upset.

☙❧

CULINARY INTERLUDE

Homeric Roast Beef

Ox roasts are hard to find outside of Mycenaean Greece, so use 3 pounds of rump or eye round of regular beef. Mediterranean cooking, even three thousand years ago, used herbs like thyme, sage, and rosemary—fresh thyme, especially, is complementary.

In a mortar, crush three cloves of garlic and mash with a handful of fresh thyme and a dollop of olive oil. Rub onto the meat, coating it and working the garlic and oil into the surfaces. Sprinkle with salt and pepper to taste. Place in a roasting pan and cook at 450 degrees for twenty minutes. Lower the temperature to 300 degrees, add a splash of red wine, and cook for another twenty minutes. Remove, cover with foil, and let stand for ten minutes before carving.

Serve with lots of wine and heroic poetry.

The Greeks weren't unique in telling cow legends. Cattle are players in the *Epic of Gilgamesh,* the four-thousand-year-old Sumerian legend of the hero-king of Uruk. Like Jesus and Hamlet, Gilgamesh is a member of an unusual pantheon of people who exist in both history and creative literature. He ruled his city around 2500 B.C., but his story entered the corpus of Sumerian, then Akkadian writing, and formed the backbone of Babylon's scribal canon for more than a thousand years. Today, it's a rare college student who graduates without skimming it on a world lit reading list, and if the epic doesn't stand as prominently in the Western consciousness as, say, the Old Testament, it's arguably on a par with Virgil.

According to the story, Gilgamesh was a semidivine tyrant who lorded over his subjects by claiming droit du seigneur, deflowering brides before their husbands had a chance to claim the honor. To put an end to his abuses, the gods created a wild man, Enkidu, who was brawny enough to challenge Gilgamesh, and, after a detour in which a prostitute sapped Enkidu's vigor (shades of Samson there), the pair met in a rousing, thigh-slapping battle. Unable to kill each other, they sloughed off their lumps, declared brotherhood, and cemented their camaraderie by going on a mythical spree: killing demons, chopping down forests, and consorting with gods.

That's what got them into trouble. During one glamorous adventure, Gilgamesh attracted the eye of Ishtar, the love goddess who wedded Dumuzil in another poem from the time. Knowing her fickle nature, Gilgamesh rejected her advances, calling her a dangerous woman who destroyed all the objects of her lust. Furious, Ishtar stormed off to her father the sky god, and in a tantrum demanded use of the Bull of Heaven as a weapon against the mortal who spurned her. If denied, she threatened to "break in the doors of hell, . . . smash the bolts . . . [and] bring up the dead [to] . . . outnumber the living."[10]

Knowing his girl, the sky god complied.

Ishtar led the bull down to the banks of the Euphrates. On its first snort, it opened a pit that swallowed a hundred young men. On its second snort, another pit shuddered wide and swallowed two hundred. Finally, Gilgamesh and Enkidu arrived to pummel the heavy-breathing monster and save the city. After a bout of superhuman wrestling, they killed it, butchered the corpse, and hurled the bloody hindquarters in Ishtar's face. For good measure, Enkidu hooted that he'd like to pull out the goddess's innards and drape them over her living arms, like a shawl.

A few lines down the text, Enkidu was struck by a crippling disease. He died by the end of the tablet. In the ancient world, there was no escaping the vengeance of the gods. The Bull of Heaven, as well as being a hero's test, was an agent of divine violence.

◆ Early Myths *and* Legends Explained (Part I) ◆
Metamorphoses

> *The ruler of the skies, the thund'ring God,*
> *Who shakes the world's foundations with a nod,*
> *Among a herd of lowing heifers ran,*
> *Frisk'd in a bull, and bellow'd o'er the plain.*
> *Large rowles of fat about his shoulders clung,*
> *And from his neck the double dewlap hung.*
> *His skin was whiter than the snow that lies*
> *Unsully'd by the breath of southern skies;*
> *Small shining horns on his curl'd forehead stand,*
> *As turn'd and polish'd by the work-man's hand;*
> *His eye-balls rowl'd, not formidably bright,*
> *But gaz'd and languish'd with a gentle light.*
> *His ev'ry look was peaceful, and exprest*
> *The softness of the lover in the beast.*

—OVID, *METAMORPHOSES*,
BOOK II[11]

The passage above is from the story of Europa, daughter to Agenor, the king of Phoenicia. One day, Zeus spotted the beautiful maid frolicking by the seashore with her maiden friends, and he was so enlivened by the sight (hardly surprising for a god who considered the earth his personal bordello) that he determined to abduct her. Assuming the form of an alluring bull with "large rowles of fat" and "small shining horns," Zeus induced Europa to climb onto his back. Then he bolted from the shore, carrying her across the sea to Crete where, depending on the account, she bore the god two or three sons, one of whom grew up to be King Minos. After the event, the Zeus-bull transformed into the constellation Taurus (an iconography that's originally Mesopotamian).

There's a similar story in his seduction of Io, a priestess of Zeus's wife, Hera the "ox-eyed" (or "cow-faced" according to snider translators). To hide his infidelity from Hera, Zeus turned the erring priestess into a white cow. Hera, who rarely fell for Zeus's tricks, persecuted the cow with a gadfly, which stung her as she wandered the earth, crossed the Bosphorus ("ox-crossing"), and finally arrived in Egypt. There, restored to human shape, she married the king and became conflated with the goddess Isis, who herself had inherited bovine elements from old Hathor.

Myths are nothing if not syncretistic, accruing lumps from other tales until they ossify, like brittle shells, on paper.

Another metamorphosis featuring powerful bovine symbols is that of Europa's son, King Minos, who wanted to make friends with the sea god Poseidon. Like Abraham, he prayed for a victim worthy of the knife, and in answer, the god sent a glorious white bull striding out of the sea foam, a perfection of the bovine form cast in ivory and gleaming pelt. The animal was so beautiful to look upon that Minos hid it away for his own breeding stock, replacing it at the altar with a lesser beast. Enraged at the treachery, Poseidon struck Minos's wife, Pasiphae, with an ironic curse. She fell in love with the bull, and, abetted by a hollow cow-suit fashioned by the inventor Daedalus, she mated with it. Their love child was the Minotaur, a mixed parentage monster who would, thousands of years later, linger on the edges of cubist art. Minos sequestered the creature in a labyrinth designed, again, by the hard-worked Daedalus, and every nine years he threw fourteen Athenian youths to the Minotaur as victims—a sort of bull sacrifice in reverse.

Mythology isn't an allegory for real events. It's about ritual and liturgy, about timeless forces beyond the clutter of daily life. Historically, the Minoans emerge as an agreeable, maritime folk, respectful of women and possessed of an almost Neolithic equanimity, untainted by the brutish Indo-Europeans who were filtering into Greece from the north. They spent most of the Bronze Age (2000 B.C.–1470 B.C.) building airy palaces, painting frescoes of seafood, and recording olive oil shipments in ledgers written in the mysterious Linear A script. Greek legend even has it that they invented legal codes and institutionalized pederasty.

They were also very good artists; their most famous fresco is from the Great Palace at Knossos in Crete and shows a red-pied bull romping through a team of three androgynous athletes. One of these youths—elaborately coiffed, kohl-eyed, wisp-ankled—grabs the terror's horns. Another, smaller and browner than his companions, somersaults over the animal's back. The third awaits the jumper with outstretched arms, to catch the flying youth on the dismount. Three and a half thousand years ago, professional gymnastics involved regular goring.

The bull-leaping ritual may have been a religious act, but there's no knowing for certain. The Minoans never left written proof that they actually worshipped bulls.[12] Even so, life in ancient times was permeated with the sacred, with prayer, and with sacrifice. To the ancients the divine realm and the profane were enmeshed; Minoan palaces are all built facing natural shrines. An act as spectacular and bloody as vaulting a charging bull would have certainly been touched by the gods.

Viewed practically, the act of grabbing even a one-year-old bull by the horns, wrestling its head and then using its bucking back as a pommel horse, is probably going to end in injury. If the bull weren't slaughtered at the end of the show, it would have quickly learned how to best direct its horns for the next goring. The calf leapers in San Sebastian de los Reyes enact a frail shadow of the Minoan rite, but a shadow it is, nonetheless. And there are still bull leapers who risk a goring every summer on the French Riviera, in Arles, where Vincent van Gogh walked out at night, pining for religion, and metamorphosed the stars.

Myths are about transformation. Usually, these are real physical transformations, as in the genre of metamorphosis stories to which Europa and Io belong. The Roman poet Ovid (author of the preceding quote) wrote the most famous collection of metamorphoses—a humid mess of lusts, murders, and aggrieved morals from which sprouted plotlines for a thousand years' worth of poetic allusions, including ones for the *Divine Comedy* and *A Midsummer Night's Dream*. But it was Ovid's contemporary Virgil who introduced the "pastoral" poem into Latin with his *Bucolics*—erotic tales about languid herdsmen and their lovers of both genders. Set in Greek Arcadia, they idealize a carefree wilderness of happy sex under the unassuming gaze of livestock, free of the ills of the city. In addition to its functions as Food, Worker, and Divinity, the cow could now add the title of Muse.

◆ Early Myths *and* Legends Explained (Part II) ◆
A Man *of* His Times

The modern religious writer Karen Armstrong posits that myths are stories about the unknowable, putting us "in the correct spiritual or psychological posture for right action, in this world or the next."[13] The ancients used to argue over whether myths were allegories, distorted tales of real men and women, or pernicious fictions that sapped the morals of the young. Today, academic students of myth—mythographers—spar over historicism, psychoanalysis, Lévi-Strauss, and the ideas of the "Rome school" versus those of the "Paris school." Their PhD theses battle under a whirlwind of academic gas. So it's fitting that the most influential mythographer of all time is also the most derided.

He was a dour little Scotsman named James Frazer, and he's most famous for having brought human sacrifice into Victorian drawing rooms. A tradesman's son who rose to Oxbridge glory, and eventually a knighthood, he was pedantic, aloof, and possessed of a blithe surety in rational thought and the tramp of human progress. These are unfashionable concepts today, but a certain class of Victorian Britons took it as a given that they stood at the apex of history's pyramid, and Frazer can surely be indulged for looking down from this vantage. Still, here was a man who, in his undergraduate dissertation, attempted to correct Plato.[14]

It was Frazer's particular genius to be a note taker. And not just as a professional secretary or stenographer, but rather as a human filing cabinet. He loved classifications, lists, and categories, and, like many of his contemporaries in the budding social sciences, he felt compelled to impose this sense of order on his subjects. He favored a "comparative approach" that mixed anecdotes from wildly dissimilar societies and time periods, stirred them with presumptions, and then plucked whopping generalizations out of the logical soup. He also had a caustic wit, like Gibbon, which makes him even more insufferable to today's earnest postmodernist scholars who cherish cultural pluralism above good writing. It's no wonder a biography of the man written in the 1980s opens with the sentence: "Frazer is an embarrassment."[15]

Frazer's great work, *The Golden Bough*, uses myths to record the nature of human religious rites across the ages. It's a colossal, weird synthesis, mixing innumerable citations of ancient texts with contemporary reports, and even letters from missionaries. From the prim comfort of his Cambridge rooms, Frazer collated notes and drew connections from the breadth of Victorian knowledge—linking, say, the worship of Apollo Diradiotes at Argos to pig sacrifice among the "Alhoors of Minahassa, in Northern Celebes."[16]

Turgid stuff. It's tempting, nowadays, to dismiss him like the limp scholar Casaubon in *Middlemarch*, a desiccated soul toiling over riddles in the dust, searching for a "key to all mythologies" that never existed. But *The Golden Bough* bore fruit.

The book, which was published in two parts over the decade of Queen Victoria's death, posited a startling theory. Like Marx had done earlier in the century with the political stages of development, Frazer wanted to map out a linear progress of all religion. He believed in historical advancement, from darkness to enlightenment under the London gas lamps, and for him, man's spiritual quest, and the road to religion, began with magic.

Magic is the ritual attempt to sway supernatural actors to behave kindly. We know that the earliest magicians drew pictures of animals. Sometimes they also cobbled odd horns and torsos into hybrid beasts, deforming them so as not to create a natural image, which living aurochs, for instance, might find offensive. These pictures perhaps honored the spirits of slaughtered game or somehow spurred the hunters to better butchery. Since eaten meat needs replenishment, Paleolithic magicians crafted clay and ivory effigies of animals in rut—cattle, yes, but also images of deer and spectacularly wanton bison.[17] So, the fur-hooded shaman, hopping through the crackling shadows of a primeval bonfire, jangling his totems at the smoke, was the progenitor of the religious empires in Sumer and Egypt.

Magic, to Frazer, was the origin of cult, and cult was nothing more than primitive religion. And he believed that the most universal cult was that of the *rex sacrorum*, the sacred king. Frazer believed that the sacred king was a stand-in for the sun, a consort to the Goddess, and the focus of a universal fertility rite. He was the living embodiment of the agricultural year, a "Year King," and was often symbolized by a bull.[18]

Since you can't have rebirth without a death to precede it, and the ancients were practical folk, the Year King had to die at the end of his season. Frazer used the Roman cult of Diana at Nemi as his chief illustration of the idea in practice. The priest of this cult was an escaped slave who, to gain the sanctuary of his office, would murder his predecessor. He, in turn, would serve until his own murder, and so on down the generations.

Frazer's sensibilities were offended by pagan brutality. But repulsive as it seemed, he believed that the Nemi cult was just one of countless reenactments throughout the world of this magical act of murder and sacrifice. Mythology is a litany of sacrificial kings. We have the Greek Adonis, whom Frazer says is a version of the Babylonian Tammuz, and whose cult, we are told, was sometimes equated with that of the Egyptian Osiris. And Greek Dionysios. And Attis. These gods are all consorts of a fertility goddess, be she Aphrodite or Ishtar or Isis. They all must die. And they're all reborn.

To the ancients, nature needed to be renewed with blood. Blood made a powerful enough magic to bring the earth back from death, to harrow hell, and to make the life-giving crops green again. To make the sun come up in the morning. The practice continues to cast shadows. The Swazi of southern Africa still sacrifice a black bull at the winter solstice as a stand-in for their king.[19]

Frazer's Year King has long since been buried under a century's worth of intellectual progress. The theory is now considered too simplistic, too pat. Modern mythography holds that, while the Year King theory is elegant, there is no unifying myth of a sun god's death and rebirth that runs like a subterranean stream beneath the sacred beliefs of peoples from across the breadth of the classical world. But it's hard to ignore the persistent themes of the sun god, his bull imagery, his consort the earth, his ritual death, and rebirth.

One of the most vivid is the cult of Cybele and Attis. Cybele was the great earth mother of Anatolia, very likely the same as the sumptuous-breasted figure from Çatalhöyük. To prevent her son and lover, Attis, from marrying someone else, she made him castrate himself. The boy then died. Bereft, she brought the young man back to life, and their cult, which had spread as far as Rome during the Republic, was infamous for its raucous festivals, its transvestite eunuch priests, its reputation for orgies, and for its taurobolium, or bull sacrifice.

Not long after Hadrian built his wall, the taurobolium became the Roman fashion of the day. Unlike traditional bull sacrifices, in which the priest cracked the animal on the head with a mallet, stabbed it, read its viscera for portents, and barbecued it as a free lunch for the neigh-bors, the taurobolium took the form of a baptism. Its recipient climbed down into a pit over which a bull was killed, showering the worshipper in gore. This is now a familiar scene to us from prurient toga movies (the flimsy white tunic, the girl's arching backbone, her wanton scream, the rain of slop), but it originally had a practical purpose. At least one ancient document mentions the idea of being "reborn into eternity" through the act.[20] Bull's blood is powerful stuff. Not surprising that the animal itself was sometimes thought magical, or even divine.

◆   The Bible's One, True Bull God   ◆

Among the unpacked corpses in the Egyptian collection at the Louvre, shuffled in between the melancholy sphinxes, there's a statue of the god Apis, or at least of one of his manifestations. At a height of four and a half feet, it's not an imposing work, but it is stately and possesses the detached funereal grace that the Egyptians found so potent. This is especially striking in the case of Apis because he's a bull.

He stands one hoof forward in the familiar Egyptian stride, his limestone face set in the same serene expression we know from pha-raohs' heads. But Apis is every inch an animal. His limestone shoul-ders, swag-belly, and snout are impeccably realized. Among the museum's gutted mummies and rigid tombstones, Apis looks almost fleshy. Herodotus, who wrote in the fifth century B.C., gives us a de-scription of the actual cultic animal on which the statue was modeled: "he is all black but has a white triangle on his forehead and, on his back, the likeness of an eagle; on his tail the hairs are double, and there is a knot under his tongue."[21]

Herodotus tells us that Cambyses, the Persian king who conquered Egypt in 525 B.C., killed the Apis calf, striking it in the thigh with his dagger. "You wretches, is that the kind of your gods, things of blood and flesh and susceptible of iron?" shrieked the blasphemer. Cambyses then went mad, murdered his brother and sister, and lost his empire.

Despite his bad end, the king had raised a salient point. There's a tremendous mental gulf between hunting a bull, worshipping it, sacrificing a bull to a god, and symbolizing a divine power through the image of a bull.[22] The king of Persia wore bull's horns on his royal crown, and butchering a sacred calf was the surest way to flaunt his military triumph. How did bulls make the long step from the barnyard to the temple and palace throne?

Although we don't know when the Apis cult took hold among the Egyptians, bulls had been equated with pharaohs (and therefore divinity) since the dawn of the monarchy. Around 3200 B.C., Pharaoh Narmer unified Upper and Lower Egypt and founded the First Dynasty. Or so many scholars believe. Even that much is controversial, since our only biography of Narmer is an engraved slate, possibly once used to grind cosmetics, discovered more than a hundred years ago in Hierakonopolis. Called the Narmer Palette, it contains some of the earliest hieroglyphics we know, and shows Narmer, whose name oddly means "Catfish," wearing both the red crown of Lower Egypt and the white crown of Upper Egypt. He's also depicted wearing a bull's tail and a row of cow-head and horn-shaped pendants on his belt, a feature that appears again in a Third Dynasty statue of King Djoser.[23] In one corner of the palette, a bull knocks down the walls of the city while trampling a man. In another, two cattle heads with human features stare outward. Historian David Wengrow tells us that Narmer's bull imagery had the effect of equating the pharaoh to an animal that had "the qualities of self-assertiveness, and the ability to render his opponents passive and helpless."[24]

Well, yes. And Narmer's court propagandists weren't the first to think of it. In the fifth millennia B.C., soon after animal domestication had become prevalent, Egyptians began uprooting from their Mesolithic fishing huts in order to follow their new cattle herds. You could make a better living as a herdsman than as a sedentary fisherman-cum-mud-farmer. At the same time, Egyptians started to bury their cows in the same style in which they buried their relatives—wrapped in matting and lowered into oval pits alongside the rest of the family. There

are cow skulls laid in human graves in the Sudan, and beef ribs preserved in tombs throughout Upper Egypt and Nubia. Three hundred
pairs of horns adorn the inside of a tomb at Saqqara.

The Egyptians liked to bury other animals, too. A macabre zoo at
the British Museum houses, under label and glass, troops of mummi-
fied apes and crocodiles. In predynastic times we find dogs, goats, gazelles, and elephants. But early Egyptians lived on cattle; the cow
permeated their social, economic, and spiritual worlds.[25]

That changed a thousand years later when the Egyptians got down to
the hard business of growing cereal crops, but the cultural foundations
had been laid for the first pharaoh to step into history by equating himself with a triumphant bovine. We also see the emergence of the god-
desses Bat and Hathor, personifications of the Milky Way. They were
associated with the humid specialties of birth, fertility, and the Nile's
annual flood. Artists carved them to look like cows, queens, and queens
with cows' heads. They were, from teat to toe, cosmic mothers, and as
such, had almost opposite associations from Narmer's trampling (and
very masculine) bull—the gentle cow as healer and nurturer, the giver of
milk instead of the crusher of cities. The bull symbolized power, both
temporal and divine, while his mate in heaven and earth was the icon of
motherhood. This was a trope, not only in Egypt, but in other places
experiencing the first glimmerings of civilization.

Today, this sacred feminine icon is most famously expressed in the
Brahman cows of India. Everyone has heard stories of cattle blocking
trains for hours, and families starving while their bone-dry animal eats
their last handfuls of grain. Contrary to appearances, this isn't a cow
cult indulged to the point of derangement. According to a controversial theory put forward by anthropologist Marvin Harris, the Hindu's
sacrality is grounded in practical, earthly thinking. Harris, who based
a career on proposing materialistic explanations for cultural phenom-
ena, argued that Indian reliance on cattle for traction, milk, and dung
was so total that only the most desperate wretch would invite disaster
by eating his animal.[26] An old cow, after all, might still give birth to a
calf, which in turn would grow up to pull a plow and excrete the fuel

for the family cookfire. Dung, too, when mixed with water, is good material for flooring; even a few squirts of milk are enough to make ghee—the clarified butter that's the basis of much Indian cooking. So the short-term profit of a carcass is far outweighed by the long-term gain in milk, work, fuel, and, most of all, in breeding more cows. This created a cultural tradition where, over time, cows have become imbued with enormous sacred value.

Ancient taboos, however, tend to shatter at the sound of a factory whistle, or indeed at the click of a computer mouse. Today, the tradition of the sacred cow may be causing significant animal welfare problems, and many cows are abandoned by their owners once they "run dry" and stop providing milk. Some Indian veterinarians, concerned for the plight of these animals, are giving them hormone injections to coax them back into lactation, and so convince their owners not to let them starve.

As India modernizes, its meatpacking industry is also burgeoning; the Food and Agricultural Organization of the United Nations says that in 2006 India had close to thirteen million beef cows in production.[27] This yields the third-biggest cull in the world, after the United States and China.[28] In most parts of the country, there are laws protecting the butchery of adult, female cattle, but the spread of tractors, kerosene lamps, electric ranges, and linoleum may whittle at the people's piety. The Brahman—a husky zebu breed, shy and intelligent, and as handsomely wrinkled as a shar-pei dog—will someday be more valued for its role in a bowl of curry than for its religious symbolism.

From the distance of three thousand years, it's easy to forget that ancient Mediterranean peoples lived in a cosmopolitan milieu very similar to our own. Cultures mingled and bled into one another through trade, war, and, most significantly, copying the neighbors. Even a jealous god, like the one the Hebrews worshipped, belonged to a complicated world.

The biblical episode of the golden calf stands apart from the rest of the Book of Exodus, which itself stands apart from most of the rest of the Bible for its flashy acts of deus ex machina. That's because it's a story of failure. The plucky Israelites, having braved slavery, the pharaoh's chariots, and forty years in the desert, stumbled at the last, seemingly easiest hurdle. When Moses ventured up Mount Sinai for his solitary communion, his people, ignoring the acres of dead babies, frog typhoons, and upended seas that had marked their passage out of Egypt, decided that their deity wasn't good enough. They wanted something easier to worship, something they could think of as a god. They took their demand to Aaron, Moses's underachieving brother, who asked for their earrings.

> *So all the people took off their earrings and brought*
> *them to Aaron, who accepted the offering, and*
> *fashioning this gold with a graving tool, made a*
> *molten calf. Then they cried out, "This is your God, O*
> *Israel, who brought you out of the land of Egypt." On*
> *seeing this, Aaron built an altar before the calf and*
> *proclaimed, "Tomorrow is a feast of the Lord."*

—EXODUS 32:3–5

Such is the stuff of Sunday school lessons. What's often missed in the story, though, is that the Israelites weren't trying to invent a new god to replace their old one. The calf wasn't a new idol but was intended to be an image of the very same Lord who had brought them out of Egypt. Rather than a debasement, much less a rejection, the golden calf was their best effort at paying the Lord a compliment. Cattle gods in the Near East were as normal as leavened bread. So when the people wanted to venerate God properly, without misdirecting their prayers, it was natural that they imagined him as the godliest figure they could rustle from their mental equipage: a strong, young bull. Later in the Bible, in 1 Kings 12:28, King Jeroboam repeats the flattery by erecting two golden calves and declaring, "Behold thy gods, O Israel, that brought thee out of the land of Egypt."

Like all gods, the God of the Bible has a history. Until Moses delivered the Second Commandment, sometime in the sixth century B.C., the Israelites were polytheists, praying to the mixed salad of divinities that populated the spiritual senses of Near Easterners. Yahweh, the Hebrew God, was merely one of the bunch.[29] Nor was he always known as Yahweh.

Originally, he was El, the patriarch of a Semitic pantheon who ruled as a benevolent deity, possibly worshipped as some sort of astral God, over a family of divine offspring, alongside his consort Asherah. According to Mark Smith, author of *The Origins of Biblical Monotheism*, the name Israel comes from El: yisrâ-el. Of course, even this is controversial. While one group of scholars holds that had Yahweh been the original god of the Hebrews, their country would most likely have been named yisrâ-yahweh, or yisrâ-yah, others insist that the "El" in Israel is the generic word for any god, Yahweh included. Whatever the case, the Bible repeatedly refers to El as a distinct character from Yahweh. One of the Dead Sea Scrolls states that El portioned out humanity to be ruled by his sons, giving to Yahweh the people of Jacob.[30] Texts from the ancient Levantine port city of Ugarit declare El to be the head of a Semitic pantheon, and that Yahweh was one of his many children. Smith notes that the poems in the Book of Numbers invoke the name of El three times as often as they do the name of Yahweh. It was only after the Israelites settled down and rubbed up against the Edomites, an unruly Semitic tribe who felt a particular fondness for Yahweh, that the son assimilated the father's identity and eventually supplanted him.[31]

The Ugaritic texts also are clear that the bull is El's emblematic animal. He is often referred to as "Bull El," and iconography pictures him with horns. It was the bull god El, not Yahweh, who most likely led the Israelites out of Egypt. The Bible is explicit on the point: "El who freed them from Egypt has horns like a wild ox" (see Numbers 23:22 and 24:8).

Gods, like civilizations, have a life span during which they strut confidently through their prime, lose vigor, and reinvent themselves with a borrowed look or faddish philosophy. Then they wither into place-names. Long before Israel's foundation, the Semitic Ugarites prayed to Bull El in his temple and wrote a cuneiform epic about the adventures of one of his sons, the storm-riding warrior Baal, or Adad. Baal is notorious in the Bible as the false god before whom Ahab knelt. In one of his manifestations he was the gruesome patron god of Carthage, where he received human sacrifice in the form of immolated babies.[32] He was also, like his father El, called "bull" and honored with graven images of cattle. Today, we mostly think of him, if at all, as the devil Beelzebub. Yet he was once on a par with Yahweh.

The Israelites may have been chosen, but they were people of their particular time and geography, just like Sir James Frazer and his imperial Britons. The Near Eastern gods Bull El, Baal, and Yahweh belonged as much to the Israelites as to any of the other people of the Levant. That's why the Israelites, too, stood at an altar made of Neolithic stones—the altar of the bull.

ᴂᴄ

CULINARY INTERLUDE

A Fatted Calf

His father ordered his servants, "Quickly bring the finest robe and put it on him; put a ring on his finger and sandals on his feet. Take the fattened calf and slaughter it. Then let us celebrate with a feast, because this son of mine was dead, and has come to life again; he was lost, and has been found."

—LUKE 15:24

Apart from being a tale of redemption, the New Testament parable of the prodigal son shows us what the ancients did with veal. A veal calf was the male offspring of a cow used predominantly for dairy, and it led a cosseted life to ensure tenderness before slaughter. It performed no work, ate a rich diet of grain, and represented a serious investment for its owners. While there's no biblical recipe for fatted calf, Apicius illustrates what gentry in imperial times would have done with their veal.

His "Vitellina Fricta" is made with 2 pounds of veal cutlets. Fry the veal in olive oil until cooked. In a saucepan, boil ½ pound of raisins, ½ cup beef stock, ½ cup red wine, 2 tablespoons honey, 4 tablespoons Vietnamese fish sauce, 3 tablespoons red wine vinegar, ¼ cup chopped onion, a dash of pepper, celery seeds, cumin, and oregano. Once it reaches a boil, pour over the veal and heat in an oven at 375 degrees for ten minutes, or until bubbling.

◆ The Cattle *of the* Sun, Revisited ◆

Frazer got at least one thing right. Religions evolve. We can't lump animal worship, sacrificial victims, and zoomorphic gods into a historical pudding, calling them proof of an unbroken evolution of mystical beliefs that began with cave art and ended with Christ. But it's undeniable that the sacrality of bulls is one of the strongest (and longest) threads in the religious life of Mediterranean peoples. The churchgoer who glances at Saint Luke in a stained-glass window may reflect that Ezekiel didn't summon his dream animals out of a void. He lived in a world where bulls, more so than crucified men, were gods.

Today, the Mediterranean sun god is very much alive. His worshippers outnumber the throngs on the road to Santiago de Compostela. They dwarf the pilgrim herds in Rome. His faithful millions enact their rites every summer on beaches from Tel Aviv to Gibraltar—braving the stalled highways, paying their tithes at the rental agencies, and oiling their skins for the heavenly fire. It's a different style of worship, now, and the blood's been replaced by money. What's mostly metamorphosed, though, is the god's image. Instead of a sacred bull, he has a CREDIT CARDS WELCOME sign.

If we look, we can still see vestiges of the old imagery, usually in plain sight. Newsprint astrologists rant about Taurus's patience, warmth, and chances of meeting an exciting stranger before the end of the week. So, too, the sacred bull lives on in the modern-day version of heraldry—as a sports mascot, or as the strutting force behind a bull market. The god whose blood once renewed the life of the earth now stands, bowed, in front of the New York stock exchange.

And it's toward money, where cattle metamorphose into temporal wealth and power, that we follow our story.

◆ A Lucky Killing ◆

It was a lucky steer, pale-bellied, touched with white flashes on its ankles and tail, and a diamond mark on its forehead. The horns had a buffalo sprout—spread wide and fluting forward at the tips—in mimicry of a corral's rambling fence. That made it lucky, too. Our Kenyan host, Chief Ole Kanyare, had owned the steer since his family first settled on the hillside, twenty years ago, and it had always brought them good calving and a bigger herd. So when they decided to kill it, they wanted to spill its blood inside the muddy corral instead of wasting it in the open grass. That way its potency would linger.

Ole Kanyare told it, "You are very lucky. You are dead now, but you are the luckiest." Then he stunned it by driving a knife into the back of its skull, severing two vertebrae and rendering it immobile. As the men pulled back its head, the chief carefully sliced the steer's neck, peeling open a flap of skin that quickly pooled with the animal's lifeblood. Kneeling in the dung, the chief bent his face into the warm, brown liquid. It tasted greasy and metallic, stronger than any meat, more like drinking soil or hot elements from under the earth. Within seconds, the stuff was already slithering with clots, but the other elders and guests sucked it down. Then the men poured the rest of the blood into a pail, to be added, later, as flavoring to potato stew.

The elders and warriors of Endikirt Osenyai stood in a ring while the most dexterous butchers in the village used their daggers to cut a line lengthwise down the steer's chest, and up from the anus to its penis, which they severed and put aside in a bucket. They split the hide to show a web of purple veins under a belt of ivory fat. Then they hacked off the hooves.

"Eating the marrow makes you strong, like a bull," said Jerry, and to prove it, a warrior wearing a dusty fedora made a show of forking the inner contents of a hoof into his mouth, using a sharpened twig. He looked like he was wolfing noodles from a takeaway carton, except instead of paper, the box was a raw, severed cow's foot. "Depending on the ceremony, the different cuts of meat go to different members of the family." Today, the ceremony was an initiation rite to raise a man to the status of junior elder. "The ribs go to the warriors. The frontplate and the hump fat go to the old men. The elders get the tongue."

As the butchers worked, they flung strips of meat onto piles of sage leaves, and younger men spitted these or stretched them on crossed sticks that they stuck into the mud a foot or two away from a cedarwood bonfire. The Masai don't char their meat. They eat it slow-cooked, so that it inhales the smoke.

As the morning sun baked the hillside, the elders sat on chairs brought out from the huts, sipping at beer and brandy bottles while their feet rested in the ordure. Children peeked over the fence. Women were barred from the rite, and, considering the white noontime glare and the wafting blankets of flies across the corral, they were probably glad of being exiled to the grass and shade, out of sight of the diminishing carcass. The butchers stripped it slowly, like casual sharks.

After a few hours, Jerry handed us cooked ribs, as long and curved as scimitars. And about as tender. The meat was pale and thin, and stuck to the bone like glue. It had a leathery texture that demanded hard chewing. Its taste was mineral and oily, and toasted with cedar. It had something of sweetmeats in it, made strange by a wooden resilience. It hurt the teeth.

Over the course of the morning, dusty, bony-kneed Masai emerged from the green, drawn by the black brume rising from the bonfire, over the tall grass and thornbushes. They smiled and shook hands, and ate brisket off the spit, wiping their fingers on sage leaves. Potato-blood stew, called monono, frothed pink in an iron crock. Some of these guests had been walking since daybreak, braving miles of mosquitoes, brush, and dry flood beds, rutted and stony. Masai are accomplished walkers, but they wouldn't have undertaken the journey without the expectation of ballast for their stomachs. And they wouldn't have walked all that way for porridge. It was beef that spurred their heels. Or elevated them.

The most exuberant act known to the human torso is that of hopping. We're not well built for it; our joints are too brittle, our feet too thin. Hopping is an expenditure of energy that calls on strange, hidden sinews and confidence in the knees. It costs us to do it, and since the movement is entirely vertical, it doesn't get us anywhere. Except, very briefly, up.

After the Masai consume a roast steer, the younger warriors vent their satisfaction by hopping, extremely high, and in a row. It's a show repeated for tourists at the luxury tent camps in the Mara, usually between buffet service and aperitifs in the Safari Bar. But that afternoon in Endikirt Osenyai, the warriors hopped for fun. Lined up in their shukas, with their sandals pressed against the packed dirt in the corral, they chanted and leaped, their beaded necklaces whirling around their necks, their swords banging on their hips. They didn't quite manage synchronicity—there was a smack of Mexican wave to the event—but it was impressive. Masai, even when weighted with steak, can attain a prodigious elevation. Especially when weighted with steak. For these men were hopping with the sheer pleasure of having gorged.

THE BROWN BULL
of ULSTER

Wealth and Honor:
400 B.C.–A.D. 1500

◆ King Servius Tullius Strikes Gold ◆

Cu is what the Anglo-Saxons called her. The Vikings spoke of a *kyr* in the barn, while to the Dark Age Germans she was *kuo*. Further back, the Greek used the word *bous* and while in Sanskrit it was *gaus*. The Sumerians knew her as *gu*—a word that even a mush-tongued infant today might understand as meaning "cow." Reconstructions of a Proto-Indo-European language suggest the word *gwous* might have first formed on our early ancestors' lips as an attempt at lowing. Whichever wise old hominid coined the first noise signifying cow, modern linguists figure it is likely to have sounded something like the word English speakers use today.

The Latin for "cattle" is *pecu*, a word from which we derive "pecuniary," meaning money, and "peculiar," meaning distinct. There's a story to this. According to Livy, the most lyrical of Roman historians, there was a boy named Servius Tullius whose head appeared wreathed with fire whenever he fell asleep. The queen of Rome saw this miracle and at once brought the boy to the royal palace to be raised as a prince, saying that he would be "a light to us in trouble" and a "source of measureless glory to the State and to ourselves." Despite his lowly origin (he may have been a slave), Servius Tullius inherited the throne.

The legend says that he built Rome's first great city wall and the Capitoline temple to Jupiter. He took the first census, introduced direct taxation, and rewrote the constitution. Most important, he struck Rome's first coinage.

Before the new mint, Romans used the barter system, with an agreed-upon exchange rate that one cow would equal ten sheep. At this point, Latin had no word for "money," so with the king's innovation, one had to be adopted. The result was *pecunia*, from *pecu*, cow. Cattle, therefore, represented personal property to the Romans, or things that were distinct (or peculiar) from public goods like common grazing land or the public roads they were so accomplished at building.

Livy's story is unhistorical; most of Servius Tullius's accomplishments, including his mint, were gradual civic accretions, not the work of a single royal reformer. But the origin of money in cattle was something that Romans assumed as natural, even though they were devoted pig eaters. There's no such word as *porcunia* (or *porculiar,* for that matter). It was cattle that always meant money.

Having ruled wisely for forty-four years, Servius Tullius met his end at the hands of his son-in-law, a preening psychotic named Tarquinius Superbus who, bolstered by patrician families jealous of Tullius's favors to the poor, threw the old man down the steps of the Senate. Tullius's corpse then suffered the indignity of being run over by a speeding chariot driven by his own daughter. The stage was set for twenty-five hundred years of Italian politics.

Far to the north, still beyond the imperial inklings of Tullius's murderers, the Germanic barbarians sat in their bogs and wooded corrals, and counted their cows. "Cattle" in Old High German is *fihu.* "Money" in Gothic is *faihu.*[1] It was the descendants of these barbarians who would take the relationship between wealth and cattle to its most violent, and far-reaching, extremes.

♦ Cow Heroes ♦
Rustling *for* Fun *and* Profit

On the day that he first rode a chariot, when he was just seven years old, the mythical Irish hero Cuchulainn killed the three sons of Nechta Scéne and took their heads as trophies. Then, he caught a wild stag and twenty wild swans, roping them, alive, to the frame of his vehicle, so that when he drove home to the court of King Conchobor of Ulster, a cloud of birds hung above him like an umbrella. Enflamed with the day's accomplishments, the young Cuchulainn screamed that if " 'a man isn't found to fight me, I'll spill the blood of everyone in this court.' 'Naked women to him!' Conchobor said."[2] Eventually, they had to dunk the child into three successive vats of cold water to dampen his bloodlust. Cuchulainn was nothing if not spirited.

He was also intimately concerned with cows. His epic, the medieval *Tain Bo Cuailnge,* is ostensibly about a cattle raid that occurred in the north of Ireland at around the time of Christ (about five hundred years after Servius Tullius died in the Forum gutter). The earliest parts of the text can be dated in composition to the sixth century, but the civilization they describe is a mirror of the Iron Age Celtic society that thrived in Europe before Caesar, and that archaeologists call the La Téne culture.[3] The mirror shows a picture of very violent men with spears who were preoccupied with cows—warlike, but sedentary, pastoralists. These ancient Celts grew oats on the mud tracts of Ireland, Britain, and France, but their hearts were always in their corrals. They weren't nomads because they brought their animals home after the day's grazing, but they spent an enormous amount of effort milking, collecting, and stealing cattle. To the ancient Irish, just like to today's Masai, cows were the basis of wealth and sat, chewing peacefully, at the base of everything from trade to marriage to social class. And, of course, to war.

The Tain begins with a notorious bedroom chat between Queen Medb and King Ailill of Connaught. Lying on the royal pillows, the couple bickers over which of them is more outrageously rich. To settle the argument, they troop their possessions out for counting: buckets and vessels, iron pots, thumb rings and bracelets. They compare bolts of cloth in every color, striped ones and plaids. Everything, down to the last trinket, matches equally with the wealth of the other. Hauling in their flocks, they count every lamb and ewe and breeding ram. Their horses match, too, as do "the vast herds of pigs" that they drag up from the forests and gullies of western Ireland.

After the pigs are counted, Medb and Ailill compare free-wandering herds of cattle, driven in from the woods and wastes of the province. Again, every hoof and horn tallies to an exact match, making the herds precisely equal. Except for one fatal discrepancy. Ailill owns a great bull—Finnbennach, the White Horned—born from one of Medb's cows. Refusing to be led by a woman, the bull had defected to the king's herd.[4]

The only bull comparable to Finnbennach in all of Ireland is the Donn Cuailnge, the Brown Bull of Cuailnge in Ulster (in fact, both animals are magical pig herders in bull form; Irish legends are less a richly woven tapestry than a ball of knotted story lines). Medb, determined not to be outdone by her husband, assembles a huge army and marches to seize the beast from the Ulstermen. Cuchulainn, "The Hound of Ulster," spends the rest of the poem single-handedly massacring Medb's champions. A snippet relating Cuchulainn's typical workday has the hero standing opposite his challenger, "hacking and hewing and striking and destroying, and cutting bits and pieces the size of baby's heads from each other's shoulders and backs and flanks."[5]

At the end of the saga, Cuchulainn dies a hero's death on the field of victory, making the ultimate sacrifice for his people, laying down his life to protect their best breeding bull, and becoming Ireland's national hero.

The martial ideals of the old Irish were part of a long tradition of heroic cattle herding dating back to the Neolithic split between herders and farmers. Robert L. O'Connell makes the point that pastoralists would have frequently lost their herds to disease, drought, or overgrazing.[6] But replacements could always be got by murdering the neighbors. As an old Masai named Ole Tarakwai said, "If the Masai ever lose their cattle, we will raid again."

Cattle are, of course, more nimble than grain bushels. This means they can walk away from drought-stricken pastures to lush ones, but it also makes them easy to steal. Once stolen, they have the happy effect of reproducing, so theft yields returns long into the future. Pastoralist cultures—much more so than farmers or fishermen—are predisposed toward robbery. Even so, it seems stupidly willful, to say the least, for Queen Medb to have squandered her armies in an attempt on a cow. But it wasn't. Mythology aside, it made good sense.

As prime breeding stock, the Brown Bull of Ulster would have been more valuable than any lump of gold. Its genetically excellent offspring could have fed Medb's household for generations to come. The triple value of cattle—renewable milk, dependable labor, and eventual meat—can hardly be overstated in a world where crops rot from bad magic and fickle gods, and where an empty cook pot is a perpetual terror. In the ancient world, even the most desiccated cow could yield a daily sup of milk (or more—the earliest Irish cattle-raid poem, "The Driving of the Cattle of Flidais," marvels at a supernatural cow that yields milk enough to feed three hundred men). Even withered hips can sometimes give birth. The thinnest bones make soup. So cattle were very much a good investment, a sort of Dark Ages mutual fund. Pecunia, indeed.

The rational act of killing and dying to snatch a cow is the focus of a great many other Irish cattle-raiding tales.[7] The story of Fraech, from the *Tain Bo Fraech* (the earliest manuscript comes from 1150, but the story is much older), opens with the line:

> Unto Fraech it hath chanced, as he roved from
>   his lands
> That his cattle were stolen by wandering bands.

Only later in the stanza do we learn that the thieves took his wife and children, too.

Nowhere is the value of cattle in Celtic society more evident than in the bride-price paid by the groom to his father-in-law. For a daughter of a king, the *Tain Bo Fraech* tells us, a young noble would pay:

> Twelve milk-cows, from their udders shall come
>   the milk in a copious stream
> And by each of the cows a white calf shall run;
>   bright red on its ears shall gleam.[8]

The nobleman also needed to pledge his participation in a future cattle raid, along with that of his "harpers and men." In the fourteenth-century manuscript of "The Raid for the Cattle of Regamon," we meet a band of warriors harassing a group of maidens from a neighboring tribe. To save their people, the girls offer riches and chastity, "Yet ask not the cattle; those kine have we no power to bestow, I fear." It ends happily with the warriors marrying the girls and netting a plump dowry of twenty cows apiece. With cows exchanged and blood ties woven, the threat of violence subsides, ending with the poet's approving line: "As his daughters' dower, did their father's power his right in the cows resign."

Raiding, and being raided, meant that the ancient Irish were necessarily a militaristic bunch.[9] They loved their warriors. Cuchulainn, the elevated cowherd who single-handedly defends his master's best breeding animal, is Ireland's Hercules, her heroic icon. Today, a statue of the dying hero stands in the General Post Office in Dublin, as a memorial to the 1916 Easter Uprising in which a small group of rebels died, gallant and suicidal, in the name of national independence. It's not always bulls that make a strong blood sacrifice.

↭

CULINARY INTERLUDE
Prophecy Broth

In the *Book of the Dun Cow,* there's a recipe the ancient Irish used to identify a new king. It reads, "A white bull was killed and a man . . . drank of the broth; and a spell of truth was chanted over him. . . . [so] he would see [in a dream] . . . the man who should be made king." A simple beef broth is an easy dish, but a heartier flavor can be elicited by taking the trouble to first roast the bones.

Bake 5 pounds of short ribs in a roasting pan at 450 degrees for half an hour. Add four chopped onions and carrots and return to the oven for another thirty minutes. Remove bones and vegetables and place in a large pot with a handful of garlic cloves, bay leaves, and seasonings to taste. Add scrapings from the roasting pan and cover with water. Boil for about four hours, adding more water if necessary, then strain through a cheesecloth, refrigerate overnight, and scrape away the fatty crust. The color should be that of nut brown ale. The marrowy flavor should be dense and full.

Serve hot with a dollop of sweet sherry, or use as a base for stews, like the Dun Cow dish above. Fresh broth is also integral to mixing a Bullshot—a hangover cure made of one part vodka to two parts beef broth, with a dash of Worcestershire, Tabasco, ground pepper, and the juice from half a lemon.

There's a long precedent for Cuchulainn's exploits. Looking back thousands of years before the Iron Age, the split between Neolithic farmers and pastoralists was one of the first steps in humanity's march to the soldier's drum. Since domestication cattle have been valuable enough to merit murder. Herdsmen, too, are natural fighters, accustomed to handling knives and spears to protect their stock. This may have made it inevitable that when the Neolithic pastoralist nomads walked down into settled farmlands, they did so in a homicidal spirit.[10]

Spurred by drought or opportunism, in some gruesome chapters of prehistory, nomads came out of the wilderness and violently robbed the sedentary farmers in the Near East. This would happen so often in the future that historians now view "nomad invasions as one of the basic patterns of history."[11] But the earliest raids set a standard for shock. Since they most likely happened before the domestication of the horse, the pastoralists wouldn't have been able to rob and make a clean escape with their loot. They had to discourage pursuit. O'Connell thinks that to scare the agricultural militias out of following them back into the wild, the pastoralists slaughtered their human victims as coldly as they would an aging steer.[12] Cold-blooded warfare, coupled with mobility, was the pastoralists' gift to history.

Among the cultural descendants of these pastoral nomads were the Indo-Europeans, whose languages, burial practices, and storm gods swept across Europe in the fourth through second millennia b.c. Much of their European brood kept a knack for animal husbandry, and for its consequent violence. And not only the Irish. Tacitus, in his commentary on the ancient Germans written in the first century, observes that, as well as swapping cattle for bride-prices and legal awards, Germans spent most of their time raiding each other for profit because, they are "not so easily prevailed upon to plough the land . . . [and think] it tame . . . to accumulate slowly by the sweat . . . what can be got quickly by the loss of a little blood."[13] Tacitus wrote this in blunt contrast to his bread-eating countrymen, few of whom ever raised a spear in anger.

Loyalty, to the Germans, was holy. Just as the Romans had once built temples to the spirit of the Republic, the barbarians held sacred the pledge of duty between a chief and his followers. To Cherusci or

Semnones or Chatti tribesmen, the strongest bond wasn't to their gods or clan, but to their chief, and the glue that cemented it was wealth. Again, Tacitus provides some insight: "They are always making demands on the generosity of their chief, asking for a coveted war-horse or a spear stained with the blood of a defeated enemy."[14]

A chief paid for loyalty with food, upkeep, and honor; this is the soil from which medieval feudalism would sprout. Tribesmen were expected to give presents of cattle to their chiefs, which were then used to feed the warriors. Already, the tripartite social order that defined the Middle Ages in Europe—commoners who feed, warriors who fight, kings who rule—was in root. Since only a rich man could ever hope to furnish a war band with its daily provender of "wild fruit, fresh game, and curdled milk," the demand for dairy cattle was pressing and eternal.

And so the Germans maintained a rather uncomfortable social cycle. A warrior pledged his loyalty to a chief, in return for which he received presents, a bed, and daily milk. To secure enough provender for the demands of the feast hall, cattle had to be stolen from a weaker tribe, who would respond by pledging more warriors into service and paying back the bloody visit. Violent death led to feuds. Feuds led to more deaths. And drunken winter nights spent listening to heroic poetry made sure that no one forgot who owed who a sword in the head. It's a wonder the tribes ever found the time to invade Rome.

But invade they did. On August 24, 410, Alaric the Visigoth, the biggest Germanic potentate of the time, ended his third siege of Rome by breaking through the Porta Salaria and plundering the city. The event had less of a historical resonance than one of public relations— Rome had been defeated before, and its western half would totter on for another half century, until Odoacer, a German, declared himself king of Italy. As the invaders remade Europe in their image, they extended their warrior ethos across the conquered territories.[15] For although many barbarians accepted the ritual of a Christian baptism, they often missed the spirit of the Gospels. "Turn the other cheek" wasn't a beloved sermon in the fratricidal courts of the Gothic usurpers, and if the Lan-gobards and Vandals loved their neighbors, they showed it by torturing them, enslaving their women, and stealing their herds.

Eventually, the finer warrior values of the barbarians—strength, generosity, and loyalty—flowered into the code of chivalry that graced medieval courts. Dark Age poems like "Beowulf" and the German "Hildebrandslied" are the literary parents of the romantic chansons sung in the bowers of Provence and Normandy, while the knights themselves were children of the tribes who had broken the Roman Empire. In the eighth century, new and expensive technology meant that only the rich could effectively fight. The stirrup, imported from the east, gave an immense boost to the battlefield power of horsemen, so war became a mounted affair. Horses are expensive, as are the coats of mail needed to protect a man exposed in the saddle. Whereas the ancient barbarian war bands were once open to any stout freeman with a spear and a wooden shield, the medieval fighters needed to be rich. The role of the milites—mounted knights, although the original Latin simply meant soldier—concentrated in the families that could afford it. European aristocracy was born.

Since medieval soldiers required disposable cash, it's unsurprising that the Middle Ages gave us the Old English word *feoh*, or *feo*, for cattle, from which we eventually get our modern English *fee*, meaning a sum charged for a service or privilege. Later, we hear the Anglo-French word *chattel*, meaning disposable property. This became our word *cattle*. Even though knights were wealthy enough to afford a horse and armor, a budding count or hopeful king still needed chattel to pay them.

◆ Monks *and the* Rise *of* Cheese ◆

Walking through the Roman Forum today, what often strikes tourists is how small the center of the universe had once been. The ruins of the

Basilica Aemilia, an architectural confection celebrated by Pliny the Elder as among the finest buildings in Rome, would fit neatly into a single aisle of a modern superstore, with room left over for the Temple of Castor and Pollux. The famous house of the Vestal Virgins possessed all the spacious boundlessness of a shoebox. The Curia, where the Senate met, is a mere twenty-five meters long. Even though it was the swirling, noisy, occasionally murderous heart of the Roman Empire, the Forum had the dimensions of a village square. Then, after the invasions, it sank into grass and loose stones. For a thousand years, Romans called it the Campo Vaccino, literally "cattle field."

The ancient Germanic barbarians who tended these cattle were sedentary pastoralists, meaning that they preferred stock farming to tillage, but they didn't move much. Starting at around the fourth century and continuing to the eighth, lands that Romans had once given to wheat and olive oil now shuffled with livestock. Instead of beans and vegetables, the immigrants ate milk, often curdled into cheese.

Cheese making most likely dates to the domestication of sheep, when puzzled herdsmen in the Near East wondered what to do with milk that was going bad in the sun. Rennet, an enzyme found in cow and sheep stomachs, is what separates milk into solid curds and liquid whey, and the earliest cheeses were probably little more than fresh curds pressed into a shape and then preserved with salt or brine (this differs from yogurt and kefir, which are simply liquid milk fermented by bacteria). An Egyptian tomb mural from about 2000 B.C. shows a dairy operation apparently engaged in making cheese or butter, and there's archaeological evidence of cheese making dating back to Sumerian times.[16] In the Old Testament, the young David is on his way to deliver a gift of ten cheeses to the field officer in command of the Israelite army when he accepts the challenge of Goliath.[17]

It was the Romans who were history's first caseophiles, exploring the possibilities of smoking and ripening, and adding herbs. By the height of the Republic, cheese makers sold their wares commercially, sometimes on an international scale, so that we hear of Greek cheeses at Italian dinner parties. Roman soldiers received a daily allowance of cheese, along with their wine and oil, and they carried the secrets of cheese making to the north of Europe and Britain.

The first-century agricultural writer Columella describes simple cheese making as putting a dollop of rennet in a pail of milk, which is warmed until it curdles. The curds are strained through a wicker basket before being molded, pressed, and preserved. Roman cheeses tended to be soft and salty, although fresh, sweet ones appear in recipes like that of a giant honey cheesecake recorded by Cato the Elder.

In the diet of the Middle Ages, cheese was what kept the peasants in protein. Although cattle peppered the landscape from Scotland to Calabria, it would have been a desperate person who killed the family milk cow to indulge in the momentary pleasure of a roast. The rich, as always, were different. Bones from monastery graveyards in Austria have shown, under the microscope, that the comfortable classes enjoyed regular chops, meat stews, and savories.[18]

ᘛᘰ

CULINARY INTERLUDE

Cheddar

Cheese making is not entirely beyond the bounds of a modern kitchen. This recipe for cheddar—a potentially complex cheese despite its workaday status—requires use of a cheese press and a thermometer, but little else that's exotic. That being said, the aging process can last a year, while cheddar is plentiful in most supermarkets. Undertake this recipe in a spirit of discovery, or not at all.[19]

First, if the milk comes straight from the cow, you will want to pasteurize it to kill unwanted bacteria. To do this, warm 2 gallons of milk in a double boiler until the temperature reaches 140 degrees (60 Celsius). Hold the milk at this temperature for thirty minutes. Then reduce the temperature to 85–90 degrees (30 degrees Celsius). Stir in ½ teaspoon mesophilic starter powder or 4 tablespoons fresh starter. You can also use live yogurt or buttermilk, though some argue that this isn't as reliable as the commercial product. Remove from heat, cover, and let ripen for forty-five minutes to one hour. If you leave it too long the resulting cheese may be too dry and crumble. If coloring is desired, add 3–4 drops liquid annatto cheese coloring. It may not color the milk right away, but the cheese will eventually attain a golden hue.

Bring the temperature back to 85–90 degrees (30 Celsius) and dilute 1 teaspoon liquid rennet in ¼ cup of boiled then cooled water and add the mixture to the milk. Cover the pot and allow the liquid to congeal for forty-five minutes to one hour, forming curds. Remember, however, to stir the mixture after about five minutes. If you are using a nonanimal rennet, this process may take longer but you know it's ready when the curd is firm to the touch.

Cut the curds and then let sit for fifteen minutes before returning the contents of the pot to the double boiler and warm slowly, over a period of thirty minutes, until the curds reach a temperature of 100 degrees. Turn the curds occasionally to prevent "matting." Stir for another thirty minutes at this temperature before removing from heat. The whey will rise to the surface.

Drain the mixture (using a colander lined with cheesecloth, and leave it to drip for fifteen minutes). Turn the curds onto a cutting board, keeping them intact as a single, lumpy mass. If they don't hold together, the cheese is ruined. Cut the curds into slices about ½ inch thick and place back in pot. Stand the pot in a sink of warm water for two hours, turning the curds every half hour, until they achieve a rubbery feel.

Remove the curds and cut into cubes. Return them to the pot in the warm water and leave for another forty-five minutes. This allows them to expel whey and harden, but don't handle the curds too vigorously or overheat, which would cause them to drip fat.

Ladle the curds into a cheese press mold lined with cheesecloth. Fold this over the curds, close, and apply 40 pounds of pressure for twelve hours. Flip the cheese, and repeat. And again, for a total pressing time of thirty-six hours. Peel away the cloth and air on a flat rack for three days, flipping once per day.

Melt cheese wax in a pan and brush onto all the surfaces of the cheese, sealing it completely. Age in a cool room for forty-five days. For a sharper flavor, continue ripening for up to a year.

Monasteries in the early Middle Ages did a thriving business in preserving both civilization and milk curds. In the eighth century, a Visigoth abbot named Pirminius (Saint Pirmin) fled from either Spain or southern France, chased away by invading Muslims. Pirmin was one of those difficult, charismatic men who seemed to both inspire and repel people in equal numbers. He bounced between Antwerp, Switzerland, and southern Germany, opening monasteries and chumming with wealthy patrons, all whom he quickly alienated. The most powerful of his temporary allies was the Frankish warlord Charles Martel, the hero of the Battle of Tours and father of the Carolingian dynasty. In response to some unrecorded jab, Charles exiled Pirmin to the Vosges Mountains of Alsace, where he spent the rest of his life quietly founding abbeys.[20] In the early 700s, the Vosges were less a backwater than they were extraplanetary—a silent place, with heathens crouching in the shadows of the alien trees. Following Pirmin into this wasteland, his brave monks spat on their palms, laid into the mountain spruce and beech forests, and led the first oxen into the wayward heights.

Out of one of Saint Pirmin's monasteries (Latin *monasterium*) grew a town called, unsurprisingly, Munster. Civilization began to bloom among the bellflowers; the pagans came to prayer. At last, the monks found leisure, and perhaps in the sociable hours between nones and vespers began to experiment with cheese.

Monks in the eighth century subscribed to a dogged work ethic—timbering, farming, and laying the foundations of half the towns in Europe. Chapter 48 of the Benedictine Rule proclaims, "When they live by the labor of their hands, as our fathers and the apostles did, then

they are really monks." Benedict himself, the author of these rules, subscribed to a peasant's regimen:

> And indeed, though he [Benedict] had been an
> attendant on King Egfrid, and had abandoned his
> temporal vocation and arms, devoting himself to
> spiritual warfare, he remained so humble and like the
> other brethren, that he took pleasure in threshing and
> winnowing, milking the ewes and cows.[21]

Nor can you convert the Saxons on bread alone. Many monks set
out to preach the Gospel to heathens in the eastern woods, a task that
would have been arduous even for the best-fed medieval traveler.[22] But
unless they were feeling weak or especially sick, Benedictine monks
were proscribed from eating meat. Only twice a year, in the days between Christmas and Epiphany and between Easter and Pentecost, was
vegetarianism relaxed, and even then meat eaters had to sit at another
table, "lest the purity of those who abstain be sullied by the purity of
the meat-eaters."[23]

Cheese filled the rumbling gap. From the accounts ledgers of the
period, we know that the monks at St-Germain-des-Pres collected
twelve thousand kilograms of cheese per year as rent from their ten-
ants. Charlemagne taxed a bishop two full cartloads of cheese, and a
monastery at Staffelsee had, at one moment, forty great cheeses in its
storehouse.[24] Cheese was at the center of the monastic economy and
diet. In a twist on the old saw about Inuit words for snow, the monks
in Cluny, who were bound by an oath of silence, spoke in a sign language that used dozens of different gestures to denote cheese.[25]

Over the centuries, monks became Europe's master cheese makers.
The Munster brethren used milk from cows that had grazed on mountain flowers and on the stubble of mown, midsummer hay. After pressing the curds, they ripened the huge blocks in damp caves that riddled
the mountains near their monastery, washing them every few days in
brine to preserve them from the less wholesome sort of rot, but still

cultivating a muscular pungency due to the subterranean damp. Firmer than brie, but with a yielding, salty rind the color of brick, Munster cheese still has a whipcrack tanginess and a perfume charitably described as penetrating. It's delicious on a lightly toasted baguette, sprinkled with dry-fried fennel, and braced with lots of ice-cold Alsatian Gewürztraminer. The licorice smack from the fennel lightens the vigor of the cheese, and the wine washes away any residual vapors, so each bite tastes clean.

The French government protects genuine Munster cheese with "A.O.C." status (appellation d'origine contrôlée), making it a rarity. "Muenster," the American supermarket knockoff, tastes like a gummy relative of carpenter's sealant. Another monastic cheese, Parmesan, the crown of every spaghetti dinner, was born in Benedictine abbeys in the Po Valley.

☙ ❧

CULINARY INTERLUDE
A Catalog of Noble Cheeses

There is a universe of cows' cheese. The following are its guiding stars:[26]

CHEDDAR ‡

The most popular cheese in the world first appeared in England in the 1500s. Often it's unfairly dismissed as pedestrian, but there's endless room for exploration within its varieties. Pasteurized or raw, waxed or cloth-wrapped, aged for months or for long, moldy years, cheddar is not only one of the most versatile of cheeses, but of foods. It's also the best for melting.

STILTON ‡

Cheese importer Linda Luke of Boston calls this "the King of English Cheeses," and it's certainly more aristocratic in price and texture than its cousin cheddar. Fruity and mellow, this is a dessert

cheese of the first order, with a piquant aftertaste. As if to denote
its blue-blooded lineage, its cream-colored paste is shot through
with teal-blue veins.

GRUYÈRE AND EMMENTHAL ‡

These Swiss mountain cheeses, as well as their French equivalents
Comte and Beaufort, are formed in huge wheels, the better to preserve large quantities of milk from Alpine cattle. Dense in texture,
with a compacted flavor of butter, they're unthreatening and, when
coaxed with a touch of warmth, reveal soft hints of nut.

BRIE AND CAMEMBERT ‡

Foremost of the soft-ripened cheeses (all of the greatest of which
are French), their pale, creamy pastes taste mild and salty when
young, but ripen into more muscular aromas given time. But not
too much time or they dissolve into a runny goo. These are cheeses
for the mind. A well-aged Camembert with a glass of Bordeaux
evokes wild flights of adjectives.

GORGONZOLA ‡

Italy's noble blue cheese dates to A.D. 879 and comes in two varieties. The sweet gorgonzola dolce is five months old, soft, and innocent of pretense. Mountain gorgonzola, or stagionato, is altogether
firmer and hefts a sharper, spicier punch.

FONTINA VAL D'AOSTA ‡

Italy's answer to the French and Swiss Alpine cheeses, it's sweeter
than Gruyère and Comte. According to Luke, it's also been made for
more than seven hundred years, ranking it among Europe's most
venerable styles. But it's not as venerable as its countryman . . .

PARMIGIANO REGGIANO ‡

The ancient Romans may have known this hard cheese, and although they didn't shave it over linguini, they surely would have

aged it until it was crumbly, golden, and rich. Today, large wheels of it are kept unmolested for at least a year, but the best are aged for three. Real Parmigiano Reggiano—not the stuff in the shaker box—is considered by some cognoscenti to be the most complex and satisfying of all cheeses.

GOUDA ♰

This semisoft Dutch standard is encased in colorful wax, and the young versions taste mild and milky. Aged Gouda is, however, a revelation. "The natural milk sugars concentrate during aging," says Luke. "This produces a hard, complex cheese with decidedly sweet flavor." Herbs like garlic, cumin, and even nettles are sometimes added for zest. The older varieties are often marked by black wax and are ideal for grating.

TALEGGIO ♰

Like Muenster and Belgian Chimay, this is a prince among washed-rind cheeses. Defensively pungent on the outside, the yielding interior is as smooth and sweet as fresh cream, but infinitely more interesting.

♦ A Medieval Banquet ♦

To Benedictine monks, the forbiddance of meat was a test. It was meant to break their enslavement to worldly appetites, to free the will for a loftier communion than with the palate. Or indeed with the bedsheets. Between the twin prohibitions on sex and meat eating, it's curious to note which one is still alive among Catholic clergymen, and which one passed away seven hundred years ago, given up as too unnatural.

Medieval monks, of course, were cattle people, the younger sons of the same old families that had once raided each other's corrals in the pagan forests. Being educated men, they also had an eye for loopholes. For instance, the monks at St. Albans monastery in England kept a special dining room next to the infirmary, reserving it for their sluggard brothers who needed a taste of meat as a bracer when they felt too weak to carry out their duties—meat justified as medicine.

By the fourteenth century, the monks' natural appetites had mostly done away with Benedict's vegetarian experiment. From a 1338 food budget at the Hospitaler monastery at Commanderie de Saliers, we see that the senior brothers, the preceptors, spent 58 percent of their annual lunch money, approximately 120 sous, on meat. Plowmen in the same community bought 10 sous worth of meat, devoting a mere 12 percent of their funds to the delights of flesh. The poor still depended on cheese.[27]

But for the rich, the fourteenth century marked a return in Christendom to the Roman ideals of gastronomy that had long ago been tossed—like science, drama, and medicine—into the cultural privy. Cookbooks returned after a thousand-year absence. So did cinnamon and ginger. In 1390, Richard II's personal chef wrote *The Forme of Cury,* a vellum scroll in which olive oil makes its English language debut. He stole most of his recipes from an earlier French book called *Viandier,* written by Charles V's chef, Taillevent. What's striking about both manuscripts is their emphasis on "made" dishes, meaning accompaniments to simple roasts. These take the form of lumpy soups, sauces, and gravies designed to be eaten with game birds and haunches of livestock and venison. In this, they're different from the small, busy plates that were shared, like tapas, in classical times, but the flavors, which would strike the modern palate as clashing violently, come straight from the Roman celebrity chef Apicius. Salted meat is stewed in sweet wine with grapes, honey is lashed out by the gallon, and everything sits under a choking cloud of nutmeg.

Of the 196 recipes in *The Forme of Cury,* 15 percent feature poultry, 13 percent include pork, and only 3 percent include beef.[28] This would suggest that cattle played less of a cook-pot role in fourteenth-century society than they did as living workers and milkers. But another picture emerges from Taillevent's *Ménagie de Paris*, a homemaker's guide the great chef wrote upon marrying a young woman who didn't know a *bourblier* from a *paupiette*. In it, he suggests a menu for a formal dinner. The first course is black puddings, sausages, something called "force-meat," and veal pies stuffed with beef marrow. The second dish, along with eel broth and strained beans, is "coarse meats" of mutton and beef. The third course boasts roast veal. The fifth, rissoles. Dessert is rich with sugared milk. Of the six platters that Taillevent thought imperative for polite dining, only the fish course lacks an emphasis on the cow.

ᚐᚑ ᚑᚔ

CULINARY INTERLUDE

Beef y-Stywyd, or the Ribs of Henry IV

In the fifteenth-century *Harleian Manuscripts*, there's a description of Henry IV's coronation feast, in which he dines flanked by the Sword of Mercy, the Sword of Justice, and seventeen bishops—perhaps the better to justify him deposing and imprisoning his predecessor. The same text includes a recipe for stewed beef ribs, one that Henry may have enjoyed while Richard II starved in the Tower. It begins: "Take fayre beef of þe rybbys of þe fore quarterys, an smyte in fayre pecys, an wasche þe beef in-to a fayre potte."[29]

Allowing a few nods to modernity, brown 4 pounds of short ribs, seasoning them heavily with salt and pepper. Place them in a large pot with two minced onions, ¾ cup of chopped, fresh parsley, a tablespoon each of cinnamon, cloves, saffron, and ½ cup of white raisins. Add a cup of sweet white wine, a dash of white wine vinegar, and cover the meat with water. The recipe also calls for sandalwood, but since this is mostly used today for incense, it's best omitted. Bring to a boil and then simmer on a low heat for three hours. Serve with crusty granary bread, roasted buttered parsnips, and sprouts. The unexpected but hearty marriage of aromatic spices, strong beef, and sweet sauce makes for a nourishing winter meal.

♦ Cow Villains ♦
The Reivers

In 989, Gunbald, Archbishop of Bordeaux, summoned a synod of bishops to declare, "an anathema against anyone robs a peasant or any other poor person of a sheep, ox, ass, cow, goat, or pig."[30] It was a bleat in the wilderness. Livestock, and cattle most of all, remained the most important form of wealth in Europe for the better part of a thousand years, and wealth has always invited one consequence (apart from flattery). Despite the pleas of churchmen like Gunbald, and the edicts of reformers like Benedict, the cattle-raiding instincts of the old Celtic and Germanic warriors flared up, like a hereditary fever, again and again until the rise of the centralized state.

The worst hotbed for cattle robbery from the thirteenth to the sixteenth centuries was in the border counties of England and Scotland, where eight hundred years earlier the last garrisons on Hadrian's Wall had thrown up their hands and retreated into the mists of history. During the seesaw wars between the English and Scots, armies of both sides had spoiled the countryside for peaceful farming. Cumbria, Northumberland, Dumfries and Galloway, and the Scottish Borders were a lawless war zone only fit for herding shaggy highland longhorns. Even this was a murderous occupation. Families like the Armstrongs, the Kerrs, the Nixons, and the Grahams made a habit of "reiving," cattle raiding their neighbors on both sides of the border.

Over a period of three hundred years, the Border Reivers crisscrossed the mossy hills, swaggering with weaponry, and capped by their infamous "steel bonnets." They feuded and kidnapped and burned

one another's houses, hustling stolen cows back and forth between fortified towers that they built on romantic crags. From them we get our
word *blackmail*, and also *bereave*.

Early in the nineteenth century, Sir Walter Scott published three
volumes of poems about the Reivers, entitled *Minstrelsy of the Scottish
Border*. They were a resounding commercial success, and many Regency
gentlemen, including the Prince of Wales himself, took glee in contemplating their bloodstained family roots. Among the traditional ballads
in the collection is one titled "Dick o' the Cow." It's an aptillustration
of the borderer's mind:

> *Fair Johnie Armstrang to Willie did say—*
> *"Billie, a riding we will gae;*
> *England and us have been lang at feid;*
> *Ablins we'll light on some bootie."*

The booty upon which they alight belongs to an "innocent fule"
named Dick o' the Cow. Fair Johnie determines to rob him.

> *"That fule has three as good kye o' his ain,*
> *As there are in a' Cumberland, Billie," quo he:*
> *"Betide me life, betide me death,*
> *These kye shall go to Liddesdale wi' me."*
>
> *Then they have come on to the pure fule's house,*
> *And they hae broken his wa's sae wide;*
> *They have loosed out Dick o' the Cow's three ky,*
> *And ta'en three co'erlets frae his wife's bed.*

In vengeance for his three lost cows, Dick rides out to Liddesdale
where he's met by thirty-three Armstrongs, among them Fair Johnny,
who expresses a wish to hang him. The violence is stayed by the Laird's
Jock, and Dick is asked to sit and eat a haunch of his own robbed
cattle. Nursing his anger, Dick sneaks out to the stable and hamstrings

all the horses except for two that he steals, and one that he leaves in gratitude to the kindly Laird's Jock. Fair Johnny saddles the remaining animal up for pursuit, and the foes meet on "Cannobie lee." Says the righteous Dickie:

> "There is a preacher in our chapell,
> And a' the live lang day teaches he:
> When day is gane, and night is come,
> There's ne'er ae word I mark but three.

> "The first and second is—Faith and Conscience;
> The third—Ne'er let a traitour free:
> But, Johnie, what faith and conscience was thine,
> When thou took awa my three ky frae me?"

The fight is quick, and Fair Johnny falls beaten, the pommel of Dickie's sword cracking him under the eye. Dickie returns in triumph to his master, who rewards his exploit with money and a gift of his "best milk ky [cow], To maintain thy wife and children thrie."

Sir Walter's notes on "Dick o' the Cow" conclude that, despite the ballad's happy ending, Dick was later captured by the Armstrongs and put to "an inhuman death." This fact is cheerfully referenced whenever the song is sung in Liddesdale.

Raids were usually committed on a much grander scale than Dick's lone ride. When Sir Walter's ancestor the "Bold Buccleuch" raided the home of one Wille Rowtledge, he arrived with 120 men and seized forty cows and oxen, as well as twenty horses. But even that was a commonplace violation. The Armstrongs, at their height, could mount three thousand armed men.[31]

When James VI of Scotland became James I of England in 1603, he erased the border and set about remaking the wild Marches into placid Shires, principally by killing and outlawing the Reivers. By then, many borderers had already been deported to Ireland, or hanged on the gibbets of Newcastle and Carlisle, and many of the rest were sent to fight the wars in the Netherlands. Europe's ancient addiction to cattle raiding had, at last, been snuffed.

◆ Ole Lemurt's Hero ◆

Masai elders have an aura of cunning. To manage their interests in changing times, they've had to rely on a vulpine wit, skirting the foreign brambles of Kenyan law, English contracts, and uncircumcised women. One elder we met, named Ole Lemurt, didn't have this quality. He seemed more placid than the others, more ingenuous. He was old even for an elder, with skin so weathered it looked like vinyl, and he spoke with the air of a bashful grandfather, hoping not to bore the young generation with his ancient yarns. Sitting under a bleached wash of afternoon heat and black flies, he told us the following story of the Masai's greatest hero.

Many, many years ago, in the days when the Masai were enslaved by the Ilarenkon tribe, there was a terrible drought, and the Masai moved their cows to faraway pastures. But the chief of the Ilarenkon said to the people, "I want to drink milk from a gourd, and I want it warm and frothy. Bring it to me at once."

No one knew what to do, until a clever boy thought to run and fetch a cow with its calf, leading them through a river so they left no hoofprints. Then he took the milk and ran all the way to the chief. The milk was still warm, and the running had made it frothy.

But the chief wasn't satisfied. "Bring me a bag of fleas!" he said to the Masai. Again, no one knew what to do, except for the clever boy.

"Go and collect all of our donkeys," said the boy to the people. "Cut the manes and tails, and put the hair inside a buffalo horn."

This they did. The boy took the horn and ran with it toward the Ilarenkon chief, so the wind blew the hair away. The chief saw this and thought it was a cloud of fleas, and he ran away in fright.

But he wasn't finished yet. He then said to the people, "Now I want a toothbrush made from a branding iron!" Once again, the Masai turned expectantly to the clever boy.

He puffed out his chest and said to them, "Go and slaughter your steers, and then circumcise me. I am going to become a warrior!"

This they did, and after the boy had eaten his fill of meat, he started practicing with the oringa, the Masai club. But every club broke into pieces from the strength of his swing. Finally, he said, "Go to Olekukat and find an acacia tree that has been knocked down by a rhino. Cut my club from that tree!"

It was the only club to withstand the test, and he hid it under his cow-hide cloak. Then the boy said, "I'm ready." But before he left, the holyman of the Masai said to him, "If you're scared of him, tell us, so that we may run away. But if you think you can face him, strike him in the temple."

The boy approached the Ilarenkon chief and hit him in the temple with his acacia-wood club. The chief fell dead, and the Masai surrounded his warriors. They killed them all, shouting, "This is what you've been looking for!"

That unnamed boy was the greatest warrior the Masai ever knew.

Not long after we heard Ole Lemurt's story, as we were again lurching across a flat of dry mud ridges between the cornfields, Jerry told us why the old storyteller had appeared so bashful.

"He was a bit ashamed to speak with you," said Jerry. "I think it's because you are white. You asked about warriors and the great Masai heroes. Well, when that old man was young, he went raiding. All of the elders did. I think, maybe, a long time ago, Ole Lemurt killed white men."

We drove on, a shower of stones drumming on the undercarriage as we passed a boy stooping on the edge of his family's field, watching for stray cows nosing at the crop. He waved at us with one hand, while the other held tight to a knotty stick. Then he vanished, swallowed by the bleached dust of the road.

A few days later we met the superintendent of police, at Gil Gil in the Nakuru District of the Great Rift Valley, a courtly Masai named Dominic Kaperu Mukoma. For many years, he worked in the antistock theft unit, tracking animals and quizzing villagers as to whether they had seen an unfamiliar cow. This could very well be the most difficult job in Kenya. Cattle theft is the second-most-common crime in the country, after assault, and a Masai, like a Border Reiver, will never betray a kinsman.

"Stealing cattle is different from other commercial crime," said Mukoma. "It's not like stealing a vehicle. The pastoralists believe that the animals really belong to them—they think the other tribes got the animals by mistake."

It's hard to overstate the intensity of reverence that Masai feel for their cattle. When a calf is born, the owner personally licks the mucus from its face.

An ordinary cow theft today follows a simple pattern. A clique of three or four teenage morans (warriors) slips past the gate of a midnight corral and picks three or four of the most attractive cows. Then they coil the animals' tails, twisting them hard so that the beasts bolt through the gate and run, instinctively, toward the nearest source of water. The morans sprint after them, probably giggling, excited for the chance to brag to their friends about being real Masai warriors at last. Once they reach the stream, they lead the cows through the water for a mile or two, or they herd them up to the hard tarmac of a modern road. Either way, there are no tracks.

Bigger thefts are easier to follow, but they're also better organized. Thieves come from as far as three hundred kilometers away for the chance to rob the Olpejeta Ranch of nine thousand head, or the Delameres with their six thousand bloated milkers. Since most of the ranchhands are Masai, they often collude with the thieves, or they snatch newborn calves and report them as stillborn. Sometimes they'll steal a cow simply because they've disagreed with how the owner was treating it. Mukoma elaborates with the story of a Masai in the dock, about to be sentenced by the magistrate. " 'But I didn't steal it!' cried the prisoner. 'I saved it from pulling a plow!' "

The police have learned to exploit this tenderness. Whenever an investigation led to an uncooperative village, Mukoma would order the people's cattle locked in the corral, preventing the animals from grazing. "They can't stand to hear the animals lowing," he said. "So they would give us the information."

The traditional fine that the Masai exacted from thieves was seven cows per stolen animal. The murder of a fellow Masai cost nine cows, or nineteen, or any higher number ending in nine. Today, however, a young man hoping to live like a warrior will inevitably end up living as a penal inmate, and as such the younger generation is losing its appetite for the traditional pastimes of thieving and cattle rustling. It used to be that a warrior who disgraced himself in a raid was called osuuji—coward—and was forced to boil his companions' soup. An osuuji today is an academic disgrace, a school dropout.

This isn't to say that cattle aren't still in high demand. A Masai man intending to propose marriage can safely skip the diamonds, but he can't avoid making a gift to his in-laws of three cows, a calf, and a ram. When we visited the Narok Teachers Model School, a classroom of decorous eighth graders collapsed in hysterics at the idea of a marriage engagement without the blessing of cows.

"If a man wants to marry a girl, can he give her parents a television?" we asked.

"No!" howled the children.

"Two televisions?"

"No!"

"Two televisions and a car?"

"No!"

"Two televisions, three cars, and an airplane?"

"No!" they hollered. "Buy a cow!"

And then they dissolved into whoops of mirth.

THE CLOVEN HOOF

The Lord said to Moses and Aaron, "Speak to the Israelites and tell them: Of all land animals these are the ones you may eat: any animal that has hoofs you may eat, provided it is cloven-footed and chews the cud."

—LEVITICUS 11:1

To the question "whither pork?" can be added eels, ostriches, and otters, all of them banned from the Hebrew dinner plate by kosher strictures. But why not beefsteak? Why did the punctilious author of Leviticus give cows a clean billing, and not scallops wrapped in bacon?

To the Hebrews, unclean beasts were exceptions to nature, rebels against definition. Ostriches are birds, but they don't fly. Otters are mammals, but they swim. Eels are fish, but they have no scales. Pigs have hooves, but they don't chew the cud. These are animals that slip the bounds of category. They have made themselves exceptional, and as such are unclean and unwanted.

Cows, being shod with hooves and equipped with a reticulorumen, conform to an established ideal. They are "whole" or "complete," matching all the requirements of propriety. And in more than just a religious definition. Cows were once the jack-of-all-beasts, good for milking, eating, and pulling a plow. They turned useless scrubland into profit, taking nourishment from ground that would never countenance a wheat stalk. They were, in a biblical sense, "clean."

Not so today. Over a period of five hundred years—the modern era, more or less—cattle have changed. They are no longer "whole." In a story that parallels the sad, tightening gyre of industrialism and its fallout, cattle have been specialized, overbred, and broken. Now, updating the ancient strictures against unclean meat, we're told that our hamburgers are mad. This is the story of how they got that way.

4

GENE POOLS
AND PAINT POTS

The Birth of Modernity:
The Sixteenth to
Nineteenth Centuries

◆ A Perfect Teat ◆
Dutch Milkers

Voltaire called it neither holy, nor Roman. But the Holy Roman Empire was at least imperial. In the sixteenth century the Hapsburg emperor Charles V (Carlos I of Spain) ruled over the largest plurality of Europeans—the people of Spain, Austria, Holland, chunks of France and Italy, Hungary, and Bohemia—as well as American colonies that fairly spouted bullion. When he abdicated in 1556, his empire split in two, with the Holy Roman Empire passing to his brother Ferdinand, and his son, Philip II, taking Spain, Naples, America, and the rich, populous provinces of the Netherlands.

Under Philip, the Netherlands got messy. The Eighty Years War between Spain and a revolving constellation of Dutch cities and provinces was a religious-political nightmare, in the middle of which lay the massive rift caused by the Reformation. Protestantism, or its specifically Dutch Calvinist flavor, was at the war's heart. For nearly a century, the lowlands were wracked with sieges, invasions, massacres, and executions, until 1648 brought the Peace of Westphalia and independence for the northern provinces. Holland became a republic, united more than anything by its hatred for foreign royalty.

In the midst of the gory years, in 1582, an anonymous Dutch artist painted a political allegory of this rejection of Spanish rule. It's not a very sophisticated work—the figures are poorly drawn—nor is it subtle. Spain's Philip II sits on top of a ruddy dairy cow, attempting to flog it, while his enemy Elizabeth I of England offers the animal a bouquet of hay. Suckling from the cow is the supine form of the Dutch rebel leader William of Orange. A malevolent Frenchman clutches the tail, and is about to have a turd dropped into his waiting hand. A doggerel verse scribbled at the top of the painting reads:

> Not longe time since I sawe a cowe
> Did Flaunders represente
> Upon whose backe Kinge Phillip rode
> As being malecontnt.

This crude allegory isn't the only example of the Dutch representing themselves with a milk cow. Around the time that the ink was being blotted on the Treaty of Westphalia, the Dutch landscape master Aelbert Cuyp painted *The Dairy Maid*. Its ostensible subject is a rosy blond milkmaid filling a set of enormous jugs, but the painter isn't much concerned with her. His real subject is a pair of cows—placid, useful, and resolutely Dutch. Cuyp made a fetish of dairy cows. In *A Distant View of Dordrecht, with a Milkmaid and Four Cows*, he loads the canvas with them. They're enormous, even monumental, with great angular bones and bellies puffed like the sails of Holland's growing colonial fleet.

The explicit identification of a budding nation with a dairy cow is something new in sixteenth- and seventeenth-century Europe. The

Dutch, in whom Calvinism had yet to fully root, needed to distinguish themselves from their Catholic, Hapsburg enemies. In 1500, there was, as yet, no conception of a nation-state. There were princes and religious orders and guilds. There were feudal allegiances. But by the end of the sixteenth century, the religious splintering of Europe between Catholic and Protestant was complete. A burgher in Utrecht no longer had reason to view himself as a member of greater Christendom, or as a loyal subject of a court in faraway Castile. Protestantism told him he didn't need priests to interpret metaphysical truths. Eighty years of war had sapped his allegiance to unseen royalty. A republican government assured him that he and his tradesman friends, not some ruffled duke on a warhorse, could wield political power. But the new nation was fragile. They needed ideals around which to rally. They needed something to make them feel different from Austrians and Walloons.

One of these ideals was good agriculture. The Netherlands has a deeply swampy geography, unworkable to any but the most dedicated and ingenious farmers. As far back as 500 B.C., people had constructed artificial hills to escape the floods, and in the Middle Ages, the Dutch had tackled their water problem with an eye to solving it permanently. They built windmills for drainage, and dykes to hold the water out of reclaimed soil. The new farmland was wonderfully fertile, and the idea that human ingenuity could master the challenges of nature took root, along with the lettuces. Farmers experimented with crop rotation, manure application, and animal husbandry. And so the Dutch grew rich.[1]

In 1645, an Englishman named Sir Richard Weston was so impressed by the Dutch reputation for clever farming that he visited Holland and wrote a discourse on the husbandry used in Brabant and Flanders.[2] After its 1659 revision by Samuel Hartlib, the book became a bestseller among the squires of England, an agricultural Bible to the plowing set.[3] One of its effects was to change people's beliefs on crop rotation and introduce an enduring zealotry for turnips. Another was to change the way they grazed their cows.

Low Country farmers invented the idea of cultivating a field for three years, then sowing it with clover and pasturing cattle in it for the subsequent three. Clover, or rather microscopic fungi that grow on the roots of clover, extract nitrogen from the air—the element that makes up 70 percent of our atmosphere—and "fix" it in the soil so that it can nourish other plants. Nitrogen is the building block from which proteins are made, so abundant fixed nitrogen means abundant green foliage. The more green foliage, the better food for cattle, and the bigger cows grow. So being forever in clover has its advantages. Instead of stuffing themselves on junk scrub grass, Dutch cattle fed on a salad that literally made them swell with meat and milk. Complex irrigation networks kept everything green and sprouting. Hartlib comments, "They mow their lands three or four times yearly, which consists of the great clover-grasse."[4]

Weston and Hartlib were astounded by the size of Dutch cows in comparison to the English runts. "We are to blame [for the delinquency of our own cattle], that we have neglected the great clover,"[5] they wrote. People took the warning to heart. By 1740, Holland was annually exporting 917 cwt of clover seed to England, to be spread on fields newly left fallow.

The Dutch augmented the effects of their cows' clover-rich diet by selective breeding, and by the seventeenth century, their cattle had the reputation as the best milk cows in Europe. English farmers, like the owner of Fountains Abbey in North Yorkshire, imported the distinctive Dutch red and white cattle with the intent to breed them. Soon, the native white and brown English herds glowed with streaks of red.

In the seventeenth century, almost simultaneous to the flowering consciousness of Dutch nationality, European farmers began to imagine cattle as belonging to different breeds. One of the first breeds to emerge as distinct was on the isolated Channel Island of Jersey. A pretty brown animal of delicate proportions, the Jersey is an excellent milker for her size, even in arid weather that would make a bigger cow dry up like a baked sponge. This quality evolved despite the Channel's waterlogged climate, which has led to speculation that the Jersey has Middle Eastern roots. It's hard to say. But on account of their resilience, these hardy little cows are now the second-most-common dairy animals in the world.

The Channel Islands have always been a gateway between Normandy and England, and in the late eighteenth century, in the smoldering years before the French Revolution, they were a funnel for a motley human traffic: aristocratic refugees, soldiers, spies, and, of course, enterprising businessmen. At this time, in the 1780s, cattle from Jersey could be shipped to England without any tariffs or restrictions. Cattle from France, however, paid a stiff import duty upon reaching English soil. So Norman farmers exploited the legal loophole by landing their export cattle in Jersey. There, cooperative islanders pastured the animals for a few days before loading them onto ships bound for England. No tariffs. No explanations. Just tax-free cows.

The glut of laundered Norman cattle in the English marketplace was ruinous for domestic breeders. Under pressure from an angry British parliament, the States of Jersey resolved, in 1789, "whereas the fraudulent importation of cattle from France has become a most alarming matter" that anyone on the island caught importing cattle would pay a crushing fine.[6] This simple piece of legislation ended up having a transformative effect on the world's dairy herds.

Until this point, the Jersey herd was a mixed affair made up of French, Dutch, Ayrshire, and Frisian strains. From 1789, however, no new tributaries entered the bloodline. The farmers were able to manipulate their stock in isolation. They experimented in a vacuum. And they did it with astounding success.

The most influential of the Jersey stock breeders was Colonel John Le Couteur. A hero of the War of 1812, he was a thoughtful, even sensitive, witness to the human cost of the war, and he kept an insightful diary of his experiences fighting the Americans in Canada. His most splendid military achievement took place in the winter of 1813, when he led a New Brunswick regiment on a dramatic fifty-two-day trek through the frozen Upper Canadian wild, relieving a besieged British garrison without losing a single man. After seeing action in the Niagara campaign, he earned the honor of carrying the news of the Treaty of Ghent to Montreal, officially announcing the end of hostilities. After the war he drifted for a while to the Caribbean before returning home to devote the rest of his long life to public service, and to cattle.

In 1830, le Couteur complained that Jersey's cows were both unattractive and unevenly generous at the teat. He decided to do something about it, so he instituted a program of breeding prime milkers. It was so successful, and milk yield rose so dramatically under his guidance, that the English market began clamoring for these Jersey animals. Within a few years, the island was annually shipping eight hundred cows to England. It was during one of these cross-Channel cattle deliveries that the colonel noticed something peculiar. English farmers, he discovered, paid a premium for fawn-colored animals. This had no relation to the cattle's milk yield, health, or docility. It was mere aesthetics. The English liked reddish-brown hides on their animals. Le Couteur saw an opportunity.

He and the other islander breeders began selecting only brown-coated milking animals for reproduction, sentencing all other colors to the pot and grill. Again, le Couteur's knack for stock breeding proved sound, and within a few generations, Jersey cows had achieved a uniform pelt. They were, and remain today, graceful, even-tempered, and wonderfully productive. A distinct breed.

⋙⋘

CULINARY INTERLUDE

Jersey Cream and Fresh Berries

Le Couteur's breeding program favored cows that yielded good-tasting milk. Jersey milk remains extraordinarily high in butterfat—you can make more high-fat cheese or butter per gallon of Jersey than you can from the same volume of Holstein product. To dairy gourmands, Jersey milk is nectar—sweet as honey, with a faint buttery color and a mouth-feel like velvet. A cup of Jersey cream is so rich that a spoon will stand erect in the pot. This hasn't necessarily been a selling point in the lipophobic marketplace of recent decades, but that's slowly changing as consumers turn their backs on austerity and return to the traditional

pleasures of a well-laid table. Specialty milk and cream is liable to benefit from the public rediscovery of joy.

Dairy farmers are aware of this, and also of the ideal of "purity"
that's become popular with the rise of organic food. Many Jersey producers have now seized on a questionable scientific hypothesis that
suggests Jersey milk is a healthy indulgence. All milk contains a protein
called beta casein that exists in two forms, A1 and A2. The A2 form,
which is especially abundant in Jersey milk, is believed by some scientists to ameliorate the effects of type I diabetes and heart disease. The
verdict on this quality is still open, and there have been skeptical reports.[7] But farmers are happy to trumpet the possibilities of a medicine in the milk carton.[8]

They should hardly worry. Fresh Jersey cream laced over June
strawberries is a beauty in the same measure as Houseman's cherry
trees or Keats's Grecian urn. It has no need to be a magic cure. It's
simply good for the soul.

◆ "All Is Useless That Is Not Flesh . . ." ◆
Bigger, Better Beeves

At the same time that the Dutch and Jersey islanders were looking to
their udders, England was undergoing a quiet revolution. Today, the
words *English landscape* evoke an idyll of velvet meadows, cropped
knolls, and the gold-green shadows of kindly sunlight in the elms. It's
a mannerly place of hedgerows and unruffled ponds, of orchards laid
out in pleasing symmetry, of dry stone fences, rapeseed, and haystacks.
In every nook and hollow there's an imprint of careful, perhaps ancient, design. It's a land as severe as a buttercup.

England wasn't always so tame. In the eighteenth century, Thomas
Gainsborough was the first artist to turn a gifted eye on its landscape,
and what he captured is very different from the twee, Victorian ideal.
In his early years Gainsborough aped the Dutch fashion for painting
lots of small elements in sharp detail, then combining them into a

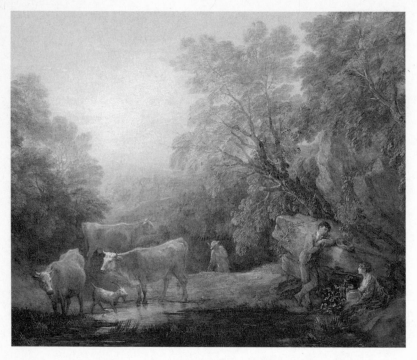

THOMAS GAINSBOROUGH'S *ROCKY WOODED LANDSCAPE WITH RUSTIC LOVERS, HERDSMAN, AND COWS, 1773. Credit: With permission of Amagueddfa Genedlaethol Cymru— National Museum of Wales.*

comprehensive hodgepodge, sort of a quilting school of landscape. But later he learned to see the world in broader strokes—wide washes of color that stream across the canvas, a zeal for movement and light.

Gainsborough first took to his paint pots to capture the salty flatlands of his native Suffolk, but he soon moved to the city where he gave up his early naturalism for a purer, imaginative art. Lurking in his comfortable garret, he constructed tiny models of hills and streams out of bits of clay, sticks, and charcoal, which he would then use to draw fantasy pastorals, creating what one art historian calls a "dewy artificiality."[9] One of the most famous of these, *Rocky Wooded Landscape with Rustic Lovers, Herdsman and Cows,* dates from 1773. It shows a farmer driving three cows and a goat up a wooded rise on which a boy flirts with a red-cheeked maiden. A creamy light filters through the treetops, and in the background there's a purple sweep of hills. The trees are full, the clouds are decorative lace, and the peasants seem plump, ruddy, and indolent.

But while the scene is arrestingly English, it's not entirely soft. A clump of rocks juts through the center of the image, giving it a hard streak of wilderness. Wildflowers erupt through the crags. There's not a hedgerow in sight, the greens are muted with shades of bark and ragwort, while the woods are gnarled and askew. This land is as much the home of Pan as of Demeter, and if it's not untamed, then it's certainly unkempt.

The cows, too, are leathery and rugged. In real life, they would have grazed on coarse hillside grass, digesting the scrub into the tough meat that coats their spindly bones. This grazing prevented weeds from being overtaken by shrubs, the shrubs by trees. Cows preserved England's landscapes from sinking back into primal woods. Gainsborough's painting may look wild, but it's not overly so, for cattle kept it poised in the balance.

Gainsborough's rustic scenes were imaginary, but they nonetheless reflected what England looked like in the 1770s. Yet even as he imagined Arcadia from his town house rooms, a more orderly vision of England had begun to take form in the Midlands. Cows, again, would shape the landscape, for one of the architects of the new countryside was an extraordinary cattleman named Robert Bakewell.

Born in Leicestershire to a family that traced its origins to the court of Henry II, Bakewell possessed old blood but new ideas. He was a man of his times, certainly more so than the wistful Gainsborough. Arcadia meant something very different to Bakewell. It wasn't something to be imagined, but to be engineered.[10]

At the time, England was following the innovative Dutch farms who were leading the world in the emerging science of agriculture. Preached at by tinkerers like Jethro Tull, who built clever plows, and "Turnip" Townsend, who studied Hartlib's Gospel of Dutch crop rotation, these men experimented and innovated; for example, using turnips as animal feed. Progress was running roughshod through the

Home Counties. Spinning jennies and cotton mills formed the first, mechanized ranks of the industrial revolution, and the precursors to steam engines were already whistling in Scotland. Factories had begun to leech the peasants from their hamlets. Cities like Bakewell's Leicester swelled and flung their streets across the meadows in a widening web of brick and cobble.

Bakewell gave himself a practical education by spending his early years traveling through England and the Continent, visiting farms and gleaning what lessons he could on everything from haymaking to keeping books. At the age of thirty-five he took over his family's 440 acres at Dishley Grange, determined to apply the latest techniques. The methods he inherited were typical of old England before the Dutch innovations—land left underproductive, livestock grazing freely, farming practices unchanged since medieval times. His cattle, too, were typical of the period: the hardy animals descended from brown, Celtic shorthorns intermixed thirteen hundred years earlier with Mediterranean longhorns brought by the Roman legions, who liked to have a taste of home on the frontier. These British mongrels were well suited to Gainsborough's tangled landscapes. They thrived on rough grazing, they were determinedly fertile, and they performed the three functions that cows have always fulfilled. They pulled loads, they made milk, and, when they could do no more, they gave up their bones to the stewpot. Farmers thought their services a bargain at the cost of a few acres of scrubby grass.[11]

The only problem was that they didn't perform any one function superlatively well. Bakewell looked on the Dutch and Jersey dairies with envy. He knew that British cities needed feeding, and as their populations burgeoned, so did their appetites. A generation earlier, most Britons grew their own food on village plots, or on the common ground that was now disappearing under enclosure. But as more people spent their working days sitting on factory stools or hauling rope in Britain's vast new navy, farms needed to produce more food, with less effort and greater speed. They had to modernize.

Bakewell was just the man to do it. A rationalist and a Whig, his life was a furious pursuit of fact. In his travels he had scorned the cathedrals and exhibition halls for the cloudless joys of science. He had seen laboratories where men were discovering that living tissue was made of cells, and cells themselves were composed of ever-smaller units. Chemists had forsaken the Philosopher's Stone for the study of particles, physicists were uncovering basic laws of nature. Scientists were proving that the universe was made, not of divine intention, but of elemental structures and principles that you could measure, predict, and count. You could explain the world by reducing it to pieces and then building it back up. Given enough ingenuity, anything, perhaps even vast wealth and eternal life, was possible.[12]

Bakewell returned to Dishley Grange bursting with ideas. He would meet the challenge of feeding the country's teeming cities, and he would do it with the most English of foods: beef.

ᴐᴑ

CULINARY INTERLUDE

Lumber Pye

Georgian-era cuisine was a mélange—a jumble of traditional pies and puddings transfused with the bounty of empire. Strange ingredients like currants found themselves stuffed into the most improbable dishes. Cookbooks from the time emphasize a mingling of sweet and savory, of meat and fruit or meat and sugar, while the use of beef suet is ubiquitous.

A typical dish of this sort is "Lumber Pye." The recipe calls for:

> *. . . a pd & ½ of a fillet of veal & mince it with ye*
> *same quantity of beef suet—season it with sweet spice*
> *5 pippens an handfull of spinnage & an hard lettuce*
> *thyme & parsley mix it with a penny grated white loaf*
> *ye yolks of 2 or 3 eggs sack & orange flower water a pd*
> *& 1/2 of currants with preserves as ye lamb pye & a*
> *caudle.[13]*

The filling would have tasted something like larded meatballs with strong herbs and raisins in a cloying grape sauce. Other popular dishes included Calf's Head Pie, Potted Beef, and "Bombarded Veal." This was made by rolling veal fillets with sliced tongue, anchovies, bacon, mushrooms, herbs, and green onions, then boiling them, squashing them, baking them in a pot with sweetened egg yolk batter, and serving them hot under a garnish of oranges.

Britons of all classes loved their beef. The rich ate it several times a week, and the poor aspired to do so. As the wealth of the industrial revolution began to seep through the fabric of society, demand soared, and even Englishmen abroad kept up the habit. The navy was the country's largest buyer of cattle, which they would debone, pickling entire carcasses in barrels that stood packed into ships' holds for years on end. Every British sailor drew a ration of four pounds of salt beef per week (in addition to two of pork), which needed to be steeped in fresh water to be rendered edible. Even then it was an acquired taste. One account calls it "stony, fibrous, shrunken, dark and gristly"—much like jerky, a modern snack food descendant.

Beef was so pervasive in eighteenth-century British life that it took on a patriotic hue. It became a symbol—even more so than American apple pie. In his *Grub-Street Opera* of 1731, Henry Fielding used it as the subject of a ballad, "The Roast Beef of Old England." In the ditty, the singer despairs of the effeminizing influence of French "ragouts," blaming a debased diet for turning the English into "a poor sneaking race, half-begotten and tame." He longs for the old days:

> *When mighty Roast Beef was the English-*
> *man's food, It ennobled our brains and*
> *enriched our blood. Our soldiers were brave*
> *and our courtiers were good Oh! the Roast*
> *Beef of England And old English Roast Beef!*

The song immediately entered the public house repertoire, where it remained for centuries (oddly, today the tune is still played at United States Marine Corps dinners when the beef course makes its entrance). It even inspired an anti-Gallic painting by William Hogarth, *The Gate of Calais, or The Roast Beef of Old England,* in which a greasy monk, symbolizing Catholic France, paws at a slab of prime beef, symbolizing England, while his emaciated countrymen starve and grovel. Hogarth painted it in a fit of pique after being arrested by the French port officials on charges of espionage.

The English wanted beef, but they lacked supply. Robert Bakewell, however, knew how to boost his production. The logical first step, he decided, would be to improve what his cattle ate. Better feed meant bigger cattle. Bigger cattle meant bigger cutlets for the butcher's tray.

He would need water and dung. For millennia, herders had relied on rain clouds to supply the one and the cows themselves to drop the other, and the two fertilized the pastures as weather and cow fancy allowed. But with the Dutch example close at hand, Bakewell knew he could do better. Through trial and error, he discovered that dung, like wine, gains potency with age. Letting a cowpat decompose increases its nitrogen content, the key ingredient in lush, green grass. Bakewell rebuilt his cattle barns so that his animals stood on raised platforms, defecating into channels from which manure could be easily collected, aged, and spread. This innovation had the added benefit of keeping the barns clean, reducing disease and eliminating the expense of strewing absorbent straw across dirt floors.

As for water, Bakewell's neighbors relied on rainfall to keep their pastures green, which meant that their land was choked with "rough courses and sour grasses." These are as appetizing as they sound, and cattle that eat such a diet are doomed to look scraggy. Bakewell put his mind to the task of irrigation. He dug a 1.25-mile canal to divert a local stream, channeling it into a drinking pool for his livestock and something he called a "water meadow."[14] This was a leveled field laced with a network of shallow ditches that could be flooded at will. Bakewell could sink the field in an inch of water, leave it for a few days to nurture the grass, and then drain the excess back into the canal. The effect was startling. His pastures grew ten times as much grass as they had before, and they were free from weeds and "rough courses." He could now cut hay four times a year, providing his cattle with greatly increased quantities of feed. Physically, his fields appeared flatter and greener, less like Gainsborough's Arcadia and more like a tended lawn.

While Bakewell toyed with his ditches and dungheaps, limestone mines and kilns began to appear throughout the North Country.[15] An unknown genius, lost to the annals of history, had discovered that limestone, when pounded into gravel and scorched in a kiln, made a fine, chalky fertilizer. Its natural alkaline properties countered the acidic northern soil that was the bane of Yorkshire farms. As the limestone was spread so, too, did rich, green grass and succulent pastures. One of the most common sights in the Yorkshire countryside at the end of the eighteenth century was a train of donkeys loaded with bags of chalky dust, trudging into the uplands where sweating farmhands hoed the stuff into the ground. The transformation of the English landscape had begun.

So had the transformation of the English cow, for it was in the science of breeding that Bakewell proved himself a true son of the Enlightenment. Since prehistoric times cattle husbandry amounted to little more than choosing a fertile cow and placing her in a field with the neighbor's bull, preferably one of different parentage. Farmers knew that it was good practice to mix bloodlines to avoid inbreeding and to ensure robust stock.

But Bakewell questioned the established wisdom. He thought that there could be only one "best" breed, and that diluting good blood would only worsen a cow's qualities. With a total disregard for custom, he began mating fathers with daughters and mothers with sons. Over and over, he allowed his prize bull Twopenny to rise to the moment (which bucked the traditional idea that a bull should never be used more than three years in a row) and created a massively specialized herd. The new improvements in barns and pastures probably helped prevent catastrophic illnesses from infecting his animals—a real threat, and one that could have snuffed the experiment in the bud. A generation earlier, a blacksmith named Welby had attempted similar "livestock improvements" and he had lost his entire herd of Drakelows to a single, deadly outbreak.[16]

Bakewell often told visitors to Dishley Grange that "all is useless that is not flesh." He never strayed from the single-minded pursuit of meat, of the guiding principle of "beef above all." He kept meticulous records of his herd's weights and measurements, marking down every extra inch and pound through the generations. He even built a gruesome museum where he gleefully showed his guests the skeletons and pickled body parts of his most impressive specimens.

In one of his experiments, Bakewell took three newly birthed calves of different breeds and housed them individually so he could measure their exact quantity of feed. The first, a Holderness, ate the most feed of the three, and produced the most milk. The second, a Scotch cow, consumed less and gave less milk, but yielded the richest butterfat. The third was Bakewell's particular favorite. A longhorn, it gave little milk but grew to enormous proportions. Here was the conclusive, scientific proof that he had been seeking. By solely breeding the longhorns, he could create the ideal herd of beef cows, specialized for the modern era. The cities would have their meat.

It worked exactly as Bakewell had hoped. When he began his experiments, longhorn cows were slow and lean, with light hindquarters. They went to market as "beeves" when they reached 370 pounds. By the end of Bakewell's life, his beeves had inflated to 800 pounds, and their hindquarters had become unmovable walls of flesh, not so much plump as obscene. In 1785, a visitor to Dishley Grange commented that Bakewell's cows possessed "almost grotesque protuberances of fat" and that the hip bones of one beast were "buried in a mount of fat fourteen inches in diameter."[17]

Longhorns were once natural fighters, but Bakewell bred the aggression out of them. They were once multicolored, but Bakewell favored a uniform brown-white coat, so he bred that, too. To boost their early growth, he left the calves with their mothers and allowed them to eat rich hay to their hearts' content. All is useless that is not flesh.

Animals so corpulent, of course, had no business pulling plows. Wanting his beloved beeves to focus on digestion, Bakewell gave his oxen over to the pasture and replaced them with horses. Only heifers (a term generally used to describe young females, especially those that have not given birth yet) were allowed light cartage duties. Within three decades of beginning his work, Bakewell had rid his herd of its milking and labor functions, two of the roles that cattle had always served. His herd, cleansed of distracting genes, was as purely specialized as eighteenth-century science could make it.

It's easy to imagine Bakewell leading one of his frequent visitors on a stroll across the neat meadows of Dishley Grange, their eyes on the mammoth beeves that lumbered across the plush, emerald grass. Perhaps he would point with satisfaction at the grotesque bulk of Shakespeare, one of his celebrity bulls, whom he rented for a reasonable price to farmers across the county. Then, once the compliments were paid and the expressions of amazement graciously acknowledged, Bakewell would steer his guest indoors and feast him on a hearty roast, awash in drippings. In later life, he, like his animals, had become buried in a mount of fat.

But the Dishley longhorns, as Bakewell's progeny were known, didn't last. Debt, exacerbated by Bakewell's unflagging hospitality to curious visitors, undid his work. He went bankrupt in 1776, and for the most part, his longhorns passed into butcher shops and county legend.

It turned out that Bakewell had been ahead of his time. The small farms of the 1780s still needed cows that could pull a millstone or yield a pail of milk. England wasn't quite ready for Bakewell's purity of purpose.

It took only a few more years before the industrial age gathered steam. In France, momentous events were afoot, and the whole order of Europe was changing. It was the nineteenth-century farmers who were the true sons of Bakewell's Whiggish rationality. They read his lessons in irrigation and selective breeding, and in them they saw the future. With Bakewell as their patron saint—one admiring commentator called him "the Great High Priest of the Longhorns"—they set about the patient work of rebuilding their land and animals in the image of the modern world.

By 1800, Gainsborough's ruddy peasants sat hunched inside the redbrick mills that were sprouting across the Midlands in fungal abundance, while his brambly cow tracks and rough pastures receded into Britain's Celtic fringes. Irrigation and limestone softened rural England, giving it the verdant greens and garden spirit that would infuse much of the Victorian era with the mild aesthetics of the vegetable patch. Pan laid down his lyre. Beatrix Potter picked up her watercolors.

No one questioned the merits of selectively breeding cows to produce either large amounts of beef or milk, and as urban markets continued to clamor for meat, farmers remembered the Dishley longhorns. Bakewell's quest for genetically ideal beeves would be carried on in Europe and America for the next two hundred years, and it continues in the artificial-insemination needles wielded by today's white-coated cowboys. Although he would never have dreamed it, his innovations set in motion the forces that would culminate in massive feedlots housing tens of thousands of cattle, each animal costing hundreds of gallons of oil to maintain, and even greater quantities of water. Today's average beef cow, thanks to hormone implants, grain feed, and modern breeding techniques, bends the scale at twelve hundred pounds. It's a weighty legacy. Today, the spirit of the Dishley longhorn is carried on by a breed called "Belgian Blue," an animal with two layers of shoulder muscles. The calves are so impossibly brawny that they can't squirm out of the womb, requiring cesarean delivery.

On the gallery wall, Gainsborough's landscapes are still admired because of his broad vision and wide-ranging artist's eye. Bakewell viewed his animals, like the Dutch painters that Gainsborough rejected, in fragments. He could look at a cow and assess the fleshy flanks, the meat in the shoulders and rib cage, the crushing rump. But had he stepped back and allowed his cows all of their natural dimensions, he might have remembered that they were milkers and workers as well as beeves, and that they were born to graze on the sour grasses of their native heath.

A shadow of Gainsborough's England still clings to the North Country and the moors. Although he didn't paint these regions, they're still tousled and craggy, and not yet fully paved. Tourists come to the windswept parks to play Heathcliff and Catherine in the heather, and to see the cows. Bakewell's animals are extinct, but their longhorn cousins survive today in the shape of rugged, Highland herds that the government plants along scenic roadways. They still crop the shrubs and keep a purple bloom on the hills, but now are paid for through European subsidies and the Tourism Board.[18]

A Victorian county directory wrote of Bakewell that his talents: "burst the fetters of rustic ignorance." The author then goes on to say that Bakewell provided the means by which "the maximum . . . food can be obtained . . . in the shortest space of time and on the minimum vegetable substances."[19] Viewed from the twenty-first century, this encomium has an almost tragic ring. "Maximum food," "use of man," and "shortest space of time" are ideas that have gotten us into a lot of trouble. That's why the legacy of this rational, kindhearted farmer was, in the end, so utterly pernicious.

♦ Toro Bravo's Brave New World ♦
The Conquest *of* New Spain

In the seventeenth century, the chance sight of a cow standing in pasture would have sparked a twinge of national pride in a loyal Dutchman, and perhaps a sniff of satisfaction in a rationalist English farmer. But to an indigenous Mexican, a cow would have looked alien, even hostile. For the first cows brought to the New World by the Spanish colonizers were not only animals unlike anything the natives had ever seen, but were the direct beneficiaries of conquest. Through disease, enslavement, and massacre, the Spanish cleared vast tracks of the Yucatán Peninsula of people. The inheritors were cows.

The man who did more than any other to open Mexico to cattle ranching was a vicious government functionary named Beltran Nuño de Guzmán. Born around 1490 in the town of Guadalajara in La Mancha to a family of middling status, he was a lawyer by trade (peasants could never have afforded an education, and the rich wouldn't have stooped to practical studies). De Guzmán parlayed his legal skills into a job as a thug for Charles V, undertaking sordid tasks kicked his way by the imperial court. He was tenacious, and he got results. For example, he once camped on a bench outside the door of Bishop Diego Ramírez de Villaescusa, bullying him to obey an imperial directive. When the exhausted bishop gave in and left his house, de Guzmán claimed the fallen prelate's villa for himself.

On November 24, 1525, in the ancient walled city of Toledo, de Guzmán accepted the governorship of Pánuco, a province on the eastern coast of New Spain. The journey was arduous and marred by a spurt of malaria, but he arrived safely at his new post in 1527.[20] On his governorship, historian Lesley Simpson wrote that he enriched himself and enslaved the population to the extent that "the rich province of Huasteca, . . . never quite recovered."[21]

Among de Guzmán's victims was a native ruler named Tzimtzincha Tangaxuan (or Don Francisco, as he was known after being baptized). On one night, testified García del Pilar, one of de Guzmán's henchmen, de Guzmán ordered del Pilar and another goon to take Tzimtzincha "back to his house and put him to torture by fire . . . and make him disclose his treasure or whatever possessions he might have."[22] Another of de Guzmán's favorite tricks was to tie a cord around a native's arms, tighten it with a rod, and drip cold water onto the bind to squeeze it tighter still.[23]

De Guzmán's contemporaries weren't always much more amiable.[24] Nor did Pánuco yield the profits that a Spanish governor might expect from the land of El Dorado. It had no mineral wealth of its own, and, being a hot, coastal province, the native population didn't flourish on being sent inland to work in the highland gold mines. About half of the deported natives died en route to Central Mexico, while the rest usually died within a few months of arrival. De Guzmán's crony del Pilar believed that, on one extended march, of the twelve hundred Indians who went along as baggage carriers, by the end of the two-year journey "no more than twenty survived, and these are in chains."[25] Since the slaves weren't living long enough to be profitable, de Guzmán needed to find a more reliable resource to exploit.

He found one across the Caribbean. Since the days of Columbus the West Indies had been shorn of their native populations. Disease and enslavement had killed them, and there weren't enough left to pan the river deposits for gold. De Guzmán realized that he could sell his people as slaves to the island landlords. In trade, he would be paid in livestock.

Years earlier, on his journey to the coast to embark for New Spain, the governor-appointee passed through Seville, an ancient seat of commerce and government that happened to be in the middle of some of Europe's most venerable cattle-ranching lands—a fact undoubtedly absorbed by the attentive de Guzmán. Although he was a Castilian himself, the southern regions of Andalusia and Extremadura supplied most of the adventurers who sailed for the colonies. These men brought their animals with them. Columbus had carried cattle and horses to Hispaniola a generation earlier, and as the natives had succumbed to Spanish germs and bullets, their farms had been given over to pasture. Beef herds, trundling down the planks of creaking galleons, spread across the desolate island landscapes. Now de Guzmán, having depopulated his own province of its native human residents, restocked it with cattle. It was an excellent business model, and the governor netted a 661 percent increase on slave trade returns by swapping them for West Indian cattle instead of money.[26]

The Spanish did have legal compunctions about enslavement. At the time, only natives who had already been enslaved by other natives had the technical status of chattel. To deter abuse, any sale of a human being required a review by a government inspector to ensure that the potential slave was, by both local custom and Spanish law, unfree. Those who couldn't prove their liberty were branded on the face (unlike cows, which were branded on the hindquarters) and sent to market. De Guzmán sometimes conducted these inspections himself, and, perhaps feeling constrained by his lawyer's training, he was moderately scrupulous about keeping "free" Indians from being sold. Not so his deputies. Many legally free people, including children as young as seven years old, were rounded up and branded. During the course of de Guzmán's governorship, about ten thousand slaves took sail for the West Indies, one-third of them marked as the governor's personal property. It was a ministerial perk.

In return, thousands of cows arrived back in Pánuco, weighing down the holds of the slave ships. Staying in character as always, de Guzmán chose the pick of the animals for himself, and within a few years had amassed the biggest herd in New Spain. While Pánuco had no gold mines, it did have plenty of land on which cattle could thrive. It even had a ready set of expert ranchers from Andalusia and Extremadura to run the operations. The human vacuum, the massive influx of stock, and the chance ranching skills of the Spanish conquerors combined to make eastern Mexico the birthplace of the American cattle industry.

From the Yucatán, cattle ranching spread throughout Latin America as quickly as the conquistadors could drive their cows. Their most spectacular success in ranching came the farthest south, in the grasslands or pampas of Argentina. The first cattle to thrive on this open range were escaped animals from Argentine ranches, and by the eighteenth century it was overrun with free-running cattle, feral horses, and gauchos. The word *gaucho* itself probably comes from the Quechua word *haucho*, meaning an orphan, but quickly became associated with a breed of rough, mounted herdsmen, cousins to the later North American cowboys. Unlike Mexican vaqueros, gauchos did not trade in beef, at least not at first. By a twist of Spanish law, merchants in Buenos Aires were forbidden from selling cattle directly to Europe. As a result, a system of contraband emerged where enterprising gauchos sold cattle hides to British merchants in exchange for manufactured goods.[27] Their illegal status meant that gauchos existed on the margins of society and occupied a niche at the bottom of the social pyramid. They, like their pastoralist ancestors in Europe, were necessarily footloose, rough, and independent—qualities that burnished their mystique in popular culture. A popular gaucho folk song sums up the effect:

> *Argentines don't wear breeches,*
> *but instead a good chiripá,*
> *bearing an inscription that reads:*
> *LIBERTY! LIBERTY! LIBERTY!* [28]

The broad lengths of the pampas meant that gauchos spent most of their lives in the saddle. Even their amusements were keyed to horsemanship and herding. In a game called "la maroma," a gaucho sits on a crossbar straddling the gateposts of a corral into which a dozen half-wild broncos are driven. As the horses gallop through, the gaucho hurls himself onto the back of one of them and tries to ride it to the finish line.[29] This game, like so much of ranching culture in Latin America (the huasos of Chile, gazichos in Brazil, vaqueros in Mexico, morochucos in Bolivia, chalanes in Peru, llameros in Venezuela and Colombia, and the cowboys of the United States), was, in its spirit and origin, Andalusian.

Spanish cattle farming is as old as history. In the Bronze Age, Celt-Iberian tribes grazed their herds on the same tumbled, brown hills that would one day shelter Pedro Trapote's toros bravos. In Roman times, there are accounts of Spanish cows so obese that their milk oozed out as pure butterfat, producing no whey. Ranching was so central to Spanish agriculture that the old spat between Cain and Abel resurfaced again in the seventh century, under the Visigoth kings. A law from the period enshrined the right of herdsmen to move their cattle along privately owned roads and paths—much to the annoyance of farmers.[30] In Spain, Abel always won.

Nothing changed when, between 711 and 718, Muslim armies from North Africa conquered the peninsula and established a Moorish caliphate in the southern region of Andalusia. The Moors were milk enthusiasts. Arabic documents from the time warn against the toxic effects of storing milk in anything but glazed pots, or of mixing fresh milk with old curds in a wooden pail. The citizens of Cordoba, Seville, and Grenada ate dairy in bulk, especially in the form of battered, deep-fried dairy balls called *almojabánnas,* and they delighted in ground beef dishes, like spicy meatballs cooked with saffron. Ground meat is a good way to use tough, old cuts, of which the Moors had a surplus since they only butchered animals that were too old or too weak for draft work.[31]

Beginning around 1050, the northern Christian kingdoms of Spain drove the Moors from the center of the peninsula, recapturing Toledo in 1085. The Reconquista took another four hundred years to fully quash the Muslims, during which time Spain was, once more, a battleground. As the warring armies passed to and fro across the broad fields of La Mancha and the open hills of Andalusia, the peasantry realized that planting crops was a waste of time. It was too dangerous to sit on the same patch of ground for an entire season, waiting to be robbed by one side of soldiers or another. Abandoning their fields, the Moorish farmers diverted their energies to their herds of docile, dun-coated cattle, thinking them easy to hide.[32] The idea didn't work very well. As history has shown, marauding raiders are, as a rule, besotted with cattle, and the Castilian knights were enthusiastic rustlers. A raid in 1174, for example, netted the lucky Christian soldiers twelve hundred head of cattle and fifty thousand sheep. Even so, the peasants stuck with their cows, and much of central Spain converted from agrarian cultivation to husbandry. But while the rest of medieval Europe teemed with monastic dairy herds, Spain turned into true stock-breeding country.

When King Ferdinand III of Castille reconquered Seville in 1248, one of his prizes was the Guadalquivir River's vast floodplain to the south of the city, called Las Marismas (The Marshes). Designated as a royal pasture in 1284, it was ideal for ranching.[33] When the spring waters receded and dark grasses flowered in the waterlogged soil, cattle could be left to pass the summer untended, roaming the muddy folds while their owners lit fires on the hills above the plain, burning down the oak and pine savannas. Ash is an excellent base for rich, wild grass, and when the river rose again in wet November, the herdsmen drove their animals up to winter pasture in the freshly cleared highlands. Given that these cows lived independently, and often had to survive alone in rising floodwaters, they turned practically feral.[34]

These intrepid cows—not government policies or cultural inclinations—were the reason that Spain became Europe's foremost stock-breeding country. Like their human counterparts, Spanish cows had a mixed bloodline. Much of it flowed from the light-coated, utilitarian herds that had existed on the peninsula since Roman times, and that had been brought back south with the Christians to replace the fleeing Moorish zebu. In Andalusia, they mated with *Bos taurus ibericus,* the black-coated savage who had walked the hills since prehistory, and from whom the modern fighting bull is descended. He was a brute and a survivor in the romantic mold. The urbane Moors had hunted him and pushed him to the edges of their neat, furrowed earth, but in Las Marismas he was free to do as he liked. And he did, very energetically.

The result was a hybrid cow with a thick hide, atrocious temper, and extraordinary zest for reproduction. These cattle spread across all of Spain, and, even if their meat was as tough as their skin, they were beloved by the Spanish people. The fifteenth-century writer Fernando de la Torre calls Castile, "the land of the brave bulls," and his contemporaries bragged that Spanish cattle were the grandest in the world.[35] And while they could survive the dusty blast of the leveche wind in August, or Avila's winter snows, they were terrible at giving milk. Also, their orneriness wouldn't countenance yokes. They were useless for plowing.

Ranchers had no choice but to let the cows range free in open land-scapes like Las Marismas. The distances involved in rounding, brand-ing, and driving herds to market became too long for a man to tackle on foot. Ranch-hands needed to ride and learn how to use a lasso. The vaquero (cowboy) was born.

As he journeyed across Spain to the ship that would take him to his appointment in the New World, de Guzmán would have seen a lot of vaqueros at work in the Andalusian rangelands, and he would have met many more in America. Vaqueros made superb conquistadors—nearly a third of Cortez's original band of adventurers hailed from the area around Seville. They were accustomed to rough food, sleeping out of doors, and, most important, horsemanship. They were usually young. And when they arrived in the Gulf of Mexico, they would have seen plains tufted with river grasses, not unlike the warm flats of coastal Andalusia. About seventeen hundred Spaniards emigrated to the New World in the sixteenth century. Most were from the cattle lands around Seville.

One of them was Gregorio de Villalobos, the first man to import cattle to Mexico. A contemporary of de Guzmán, he grew up in Las Marismas before seeking his fortune with the conquistadors. Unlike many other Spanish adventurers, he didn't pen letters complaining about his hardships, but we know of him because he was mayor of one of the earliest Spanish settlements, and he was probably an intimate of de Guzmán. It was de Villalobos who most likely gave de Guzmán the idea to ranch beef cattle on a gargantuan scale. Perhaps, while visiting the governor's private estate on a mission to kindle his acquisitive ap-petites, he pointed at the wet lowlands thrumming with mosquitoes, and at the scraggly uplands nearby. They could ranch here just like at home in Las Marismas, he might have said. It was the same type of land, more or less, and the men knew how to do it. All they needed was the cows.

The Spanish crown was very generous in granting colonial lands to men pledging to raise beef cattle, and de Villalobos's descendants were the biggest beneficiaries of this policy. His family owned enormous estancias (ranches), which they worked as they had always done. As late as the nineteenth century, a visitor to a Villalobos estancia wrote:

> ... [with] the cessation of the rains, the [higher]
> prairies fade, the soil dries up, the trees lose their
> foliage, the herds seek the forests and chasms, and in
> the cloudless skies, the sun scorches up the unsheltered
> plains.

Before the vaqueros drove the animals down from their summer quarters and into the prairies, they set them ablaze,

> partly to destroy the clouds of tormenting ticks and
> tarantulas, partly to call forth a new crop from beneath
> the ashes.[36]

Then, with the return of the rains, the cows again took the high ground.

It was a very efficient ranching system, but it had the consequence of completely obliterating any native settlements that had enough luck to survive the slave trade. The indigenous people had, for centuries, farmed this land using elaborate drainage networks and raised fields. Now it was given over to half-wild herds of ornery cows. They didn't need much encouragement to be fruitful. By 1620, de Guzmán's province of Pánuco harbored 176,000 head.[37] Ranching was one of colonization's most effective tools.

For the people de Guzmán enslaved and deported, his governorship was a wretched story. Nor did it turn out well for the man himself. He died, penniless, in a Spanish prison, complaining to the last about wages unpaid by the crown, and about the malice of a government that robbed him, unjustly, of his own slaves.

What happened to cattle between 1500 and 1800 is what happened to the world. As the map unfolded and religions splintered and old truths fell apart at the first gust of change, new nations had to be built out of the dust. So did empires. So did ideas. And one of these ideas was the concept that we could take an animal and reshape it any way we liked. Instead of thinking about cattle as sacred, or merely valuable, we learned to think of them as a problem to be solved.

The Dutch, who created a republic of free citizens before the British or Americans or French ever experimented with parliaments, were also the first to invent specialized cattle. These ingenious farmers had, through centuries of toil, remolded their entire landscape in the name of good agriculture and profit. Cows were an obvious candidate for similar treatment. The Dutch dairy cow became so central to the economy, and such an important source of revenue, that she could symbolize the country as a whole, rallying farmers and townsmen alike in the fight for independence. Reversing the symbol, on the other side of the Spanish Empire, militant cowboys planted their ranching culture, along with their beloved beef cows, on the territories they conquered. Meanwhile, the English were quietly tinkering toward the industrial revolution. They treated their cows like machines—objects to be improved with a tweak and some clever reassembly.

What the Dutch, the English, and the Spanish forgot was the ancient view of a whole animal that worked, and yielded milk, and died, after a productive life, for the good of the stewpot. They split the species into beeves and milkers, breeding meatier carcasses and faster-flowing udders. Nor did these specialized animals live in wood and scrub. New, huge kingdoms of cattle stretched across both the New and Old Worlds. But a line had been crossed. Once farmers started thinking that cattle could be reduced to their constituent parts for the sake of profit, they stopped thinking of them as complex, living creatures. They ceased to be animals, and they became commodities.

◆ The Woman *of* Narok ◆

If you want to stand an Iron Age pastoralist society on its ear, give every adult male a lump of prime real estate and let loose the lawyers. This is what happened to the Masai at the turn of the millennium when the tribe began to divvy up common pasturelands, granting each member a parcel of forty acres. The motive—popular among international development policy wonks at the time—was to encourage private enterprise and personal responsibility among people who had never heard the words "market efficiency." But since the Masai discovered capitalism late (not materialism; their lively connoisseurship for cows now extends to cell phones and late-model SUVs), they've worn it poorly. Even in the twenty-first century, all too often a Masai entrepreneurial initiative involves little more than a wooden club and cover of night.

"A lot of [the Masai] couldn't read the contracts, so they sold their land for next to nothing and lost it all," said Jerry. Change, like money, is flowing fast in Masailand. Young people are moving to the city, the haves have more, the have-nots take their usual plunge toward the bottom of the free market. Malnutrition, among some of the least fortunate, once more flaps its spindly wings.[38] We were driving on one of Kenya's demonically awful roads, the axles of our jeep howling as we pushed past long fields of yellowing wheat. About fifty yards away in the grain, a herd of zebra milled, looking natty. Jerry watched them in cool distaste.

"That farmer is going to be very angry," he said. "They're stealing his crop." This zebra-aggrieved farmer, however, was as likely to be a Kikuyu or Luhya tribesman as a Masai. One of the effects of land reform is that other ethnic groups have bought up the once open pastures that had been collective Masai property. Instead of raising cattle on them, the newcomers have a taste for cash crops. Grasslands that Masai herds had grazed a few years ago are now clogged with maize and beans, and it's become an accepted agricultural expense to pay small children to stand on the roadside and drive trespassing cows away from the wheat. With the loss of so much pasture, herdsmen are obliged to walk their animals deeper toward the Masai Mara, a wildlife preserve where they often encroach on grasslands reserved for gazelles. This leaves the herdsmen open to the attacks of both lions and wildlife conservationists.

A few miles farther up the road, the wheat gave way to long, acacia-shaded pastures. Jerry swerved around a pothole that could have easily swallowed a three-bedroom walk-up, and then we stopped in a dusty spread of rectangular huts owned by an elder named Kapolonto Ole Lempaka. He was a stately octogenarian—Masai age well—and one of his wives poured boiling chai while he told us the story of the great cattle raid of the Ildamat clan. Jerry spoke to Ole Lempaka with an especial deference, leaning forward and lowering his eyes. The two were both Ildamat, it turned out, while the other elders we had met all belonged to the more plentiful Purko.

Ole Lempaka's first wife had draped the sunless, mud room with Indian printed sheets. Chipped tin chai cups sat on a tablecloth. The sofa, though starved for stuffing, was upholstered. This was evidently the home of a man of respect, one with a son on the Narok city council and many hundreds of cows. He had done well in these changing times.

The Masai have a saying about the rich: "Today you have wealth. Tomorrow it's my turn." Despite their poverty, or perhaps because of it, the Masai don't begrudge a man his fortune. But they're not Horatio Algers in tribal shukas. They understand that wealth, like all things, will pass.

Ole Lempaka explained why we had met so few of his clansmen on our travels.

"The reason why there are so few Ildamat left is that many years ago, smallpox killed thousands of our warriors," he said. "Any warrior who dies fighting is a hero, and will be talked about forever. His family receives two hundred cows from the other warriors, and people say, 'He went, but here are his animals!'

"But a warrior who dies of disease is unlucky," said the old man. "He is cursed."

"The Masai aren't afraid of death, because they can't envision the future," said Jerry. Living among cows, with their standing births and their skin ailments and their noisy alimentary habits, with a purely physical existence, it might seem that the Masai would be painfully conscious of the weakness of flesh. But then, cows don't worry about dying. Merely and fully, they live. That's bound to make an impression on a young African boy, sitting on the unlit roadside in the company of a few dozen animals that do nothing but chew and fart. In such a case, it must be tempting to embrace a materialist view of the universe. We are atoms, this cow and I. So I had better eat steak.

When a Masai dies, his family smears his body with the fat of a fresh-butchered steer, and his sons divide his property in equal shares. Until a few years ago, this meant applying simple long division to his cattle, and perhaps doling out a few blankets, swords, and beads. Since land subdivision began the matter of legacies has become more fraught. If a man like Ole Lempaka has forty acres and ten sons, in a few years ten aging Masai will own four acres apiece. The land will be so fractured as to be valueless. Even if the plots congealed, the common pasture is already almost gone, and cattle will never again graze on lands that have been planted with corn. The old life is over.

"Since time immemorial, the Masai had a good life," sighed Ole Lempaka. "The children walked naked and never became sick. The cattle never had diseases."

"Except for twice," added Jerry. "Rinderpest and contagious bovine pleuropneumonia." And there are other, more modern plagues, like the lurking horror of Rift Valley fever. It spreads from livestock to human beings by contact with raw blood or milk, or by mosquito bites. In late 2006 it killed more than a hundred Kenyans, most of them herdsmen or young women handling the family meals.

Even in the face of purulent illness, there are Masai who prefer simply not to look. Jerry tells the story of old man Olalarok, who lives near the Mara. "Every year when I try to vaccinate his herd, he stands with his sons, all of them armed with bows and arrows, and shouts, 'You'll have to kill me before you touch my cattle!' Of course, when he's away, his sons come to me and we vaccinate them anyway." It's worth the risk. If there's a belt of the most murderous vectorborne diseases in the world (malaria, sleeping sickness, dengue), then Kenya sits at its buckle.

"But if the old man found out we were vaccinating his cattle," said Jerry, "he would kill [his sons] with a spear." *Patria potestas,* indeed. The familial grip held by Masai fathers makes even the grimmest old Romans look like cupcakes in comparison. Cattle, wives, and children are theirs to rule.

When we drove back into town, we stopped at the cattle market. It was there that we saw the most elegant woman in Narok, armored in beige polyester, in the middle of a thousand cows. She wore a square jacket, a knee-length skirt, and a gray headscarf folded, not in the piled, turban style favored by African ladies, but in a flat, Jacqueline Onassis wrap. She was the only person on the dirt grounds of the market to be clutching a handbag. Everyone else was male, and they clutched clubs.

"She's a butcher," said Jerry, who was walking us through the mad crush of Narok's cattle market. "She's here to buy." The elegant woman was peering with cool interest at the backside of a large white steer. She jotted something into a notebook and spoke to a dusty little man who started negotiating with the cow's seller. Although she was a customer and person to be respected, the Masai feel that cows belong to the manly sphere of business and social rank. Except for when they need milking. Then they become woman's work. At the market, though, the elegant butcher had to speak through a male surrogate.

Gender equality has not quite penetrated the Masai, who, like many other rural African tribes, are still enthusiastic cliteridectomists. During our corral feast, the gentle elder named Ole Lemurt had told the Masai legend on the separation of the sexes.

"It used to be that men and women were all warriors," he said. "And women were the stronger. Warriors travel in pairs, so that one can keep watch while the other sleeps, and when they stop to drink, one of them plants his spear in the ground while his companion watches over him. One day a pair of warriors came to a stream, and as they bent down, the guard prodded his companion with his shield. 'Don't do that!' cried his companion, for he had pushed the edge of it into the female organ.

"Now, the warrior didn't know what to do, and the woman said, 'If you don't expose me, you can use your penis on me for pleasure.' She became pregnant, and was unable to go on cattle raids, and the warrior was left tending to her, for they pretended she was sick with disease. When the other warriors returned from a raid, she had given birth, and they could no longer hide that she was a woman. The men decided to check everyone, and they discovered all the women among them. They decided to get rid of them.

"So the men went to God with their problem, and God said, 'They're too strong for you to fight. Take them to the waterfall, and I will confuse them.' They led all the women to the waterfall, and as they looked down, God muddled them, and weakened them. And from that moment, they were subject to being married. And that is how we came to be separate."

Unlike the genders, the cattle in Narok's livestock market are anything but segregated. There was nothing to tell a dairy cow from a beef cow and the market's cluster of linked corrals—from above it must look something like the Olympics symbol in red cedar—teemed with life on a blistering Sunday morning. Hundreds of animals were pushing their shoulders against the fences and getting stuck in gates. Sometimes one would lower its head and sprint, at which the men would erupt in a brief, frantic imitation of Pamplona. In every other place we had visited, the Masai had behaved in a calm, even bemused, manner. But the cattle market was no place for detachment. Stately, red-cloaked herdsmen, who had spent years in quiet study of broad, lonely horizons, jabbered like excited hens. Traders in dungarees slapped palms, sweated, and shrieked. The center of much of the morning's excitement was a towering bull the color of Marquinia marble. It strutted through the lesser animals like a fleshy prince, a trail of love-struck Masai in its wake. Even Jerry's head turned.

"It's a crossbreed," he said, a hungry glimmer flashing across his eyes. "It must weigh eight hundred kilos." It was truly a glorious cow.

The Masai zebu around it looked stubby and frail by comparison, their bones jutting weakly out of their taut, tan hides. Most of them weighed no more than 160 kilograms, 90 after being bled and gutted. This animal was worth five of the others.

"There's an idea going around to improve the Masai cattle," said Jerry. We had stopped to look at the most pathetic steer in the market. It stood at the height of an Irish wolfhound, and its coat was riddled with a patchy fungus. The seller assured us that the animal was being medicated, but it hung its skewed horns, and looked worried, and didn't attract any buyers. Jerry clucked over it for a moment, then moved on, shaking his head. "In the north, there are now attempts to increase size by crossbreeding with Boran cattle and Sahiwal." Sahiwal are native to India and are the best of the zebu milkers. Boran are hardy, medium-sized beef cows that originated along the Ethiopian border. Both are good at shrugging off ticks and violent sunlight, and both are much more productive than the Masai's breeds.

"If we can improve the cattle here, people might be willing to reduce the size of their herds," said Jerry. Cattle improvement is one of his numerous crusades. "The Masai have too many cattle. I know an eighty-year-old elder who had four thousand cows. He rents 80 percent of his land to farmers. He can't maintain his animals on that, but he won't sell any of his stock! Last year I persuaded him to sell four hundred cows, but with the profit from the sale and from his rentals, he bought more cattle. When I confronted him about it, he said, 'Son, do you want me to be a pauper?'"

Outside the corral, we crossed a ring of vendors selling bananas and swords laid out on blankets in the grass. The elegant butcher had finished her dealings and was being escorted to her car, her heels gouging divots out of the soft, cropped pasture that surrounded the market. A string of bony, splay-uddered cows looked up from their grazing as she passed, following her with welling eyes. Then they turned back to the business of digestion.

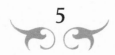

5

CATTLE KINGS
AND DAIRY QUEENS

*The Industrialization of Food:
The Nineteenth Century*

◆ War, Pandemics, *and* Famine ◆

On December 6, 1240, the Mongol army of Batu Khan, grandson of Genghis, stormed the Russian city of Kiev after a nine-day siege. Behaving in character, they massacred most of the inhabitants and burned the city around the ears of the survivors, just as they had habitually done throughout Eurasia. The suddenness with which Kiev's defenses fell is recorded in the archaeological record: a pot of porridge with the spoon still inside; crystal beads stashed in a jug and dropped in the tumult; a collapsed escape tunnel; two girls huddled together inside a stove.[1] The Mongols were nothing if not direct.

Batu's army was staggeringly large—150,000 soldiers, trailing families, merchants, and, of course, livestock. The Mongols were horse people, and they were also famously well stocked in sheep and cattle.

So many cows were present at the siege that the lowing drowned out the cries of the horrified townsfolk.

✌❧

CULINARY INTERLUDE

Steak Tartare

In the Middle Ages, uninformed Europeans sometimes confused Mongols with Tartars, believing every mob of bloodthirsty Asiatics to be of a type. Hence the legend of "steak tartare" originating as raw meat kept under the saddles of Genghis Khan's warriors, either as a method of tenderization or to reduce saddle sores. The story is apocryphal, but in the English-speaking world, a dish of seasoned, raw, chopped beef has acquired a reputation for exoticism and danger (contrariwise, in Belgium and the Netherlands the dish bears the prosaic title of filet américain). It's most often encountered in places where diners value flavor over caution or budget. In other words, French restaurants.

In a large bowl, combine 2 egg yolks with 1 teaspoon Dijon mustard, 1 teaspoon Worcestershire sauce, ¼ cup olive oil, 2 cloves crushed garlic, 1 teaspoon finely diced sun-blushed tomatoes, and the juice from one lemon. Add salt and pepper or hot sauce to taste and whisk until thickened. Add ¾ pound ground, prime sirloin or tenderloin, 2 finely diced shallots, 3 teaspoons capers, 4 tablespoons chopped fresh coriander, and mix well. Form the meat into four or five circular patties and serve with toast points, homemade croutons, or French fries.

It's important to use lean, high-quality meat for this recipe, and to remove all the fat and sinew before grinding. Since the meat is cold, the flavor of the beef shouldn't be too strong (if it is, hurry to the nearest toilet—you'll be needing it). Rather, it ought to play off the garlic, capers, sun-blushed tomatoes, and coriander. Much like carpaccio, which is simply raw sliced steak, the inherent flavors in the meat haven't been brought forth by heating, so it serves more as a foundation for the seasonings than as the starring taste.

If Genghis Khan ever ate this, however, it's to be hoped he would have rinsed off the horse sweat.

What the Kievan Rus didn't know was that the Mongols carried something worse than fire and sword (although this was little consolation for those put to the fire and sword). Their cattle were infected with rinderpest—the most virulent of all livestock diseases—a virus closely related to human measles, but deadlier. For thousands of years it had been confined to East Asia, but now the invaders' herds spread the blight through Europe's sheltered farmlands.

Cattle diseases had attacked Europe before rinderpest. In Virgil's *Georgics,* written in 31 B.C., the poet of the Augustan age describes a plague where "wild beasts and cattle met an equal death/each pool, each pasture, felt the poisonous breath." In 694, the Irish Annals of Clonmacnoise record that there was "a great morren of cattle throughout all England." But these were isolated plagues. The first European outbreak of rinderpest dates to the thirteenth century and follows the train of Batu's Golden Horde.[2]

Like a pebble dropped in a millpond, the disease annihilated cattle herds first in Hungary and Austria, then Germany, Italy, France, and England, where a majority of the country's cows probably died.[3] In Scotland it gave an unexpected boost to the cause of Scottish independence, when, in 1319, the oxen used by Edward II to besiege the town of Berwick fell ill. The oxen perished, and, unable to pull his engines, Edward retreated. Berwick's cows must have died, too.

Rinderpest is a quicksilver sickness. It passes—indirectly, if necessary—between hosts by means of tears, saliva, nasal secretions, urine, and feces. Every type of bodily fluid and tissue is infectious, and because it needs three to fifteen days to incubate, a carrier animal can walk a long distance and infect a great many others before it succumbs.[4]

A nineteenth-century British witness observed:

> *After the fourth day [since the fever is observed] . . .*
> *the constitution is thoroughly invaded. Then ensue*
> *the urgent symptoms,—the drooping head, the*
> *hanging ears, the distressed look, the failing pulse,*
> *the oppressed breathing, the discharge from the eyes,*
> *nose, and mouth, the eruption of the skin, the foetid*
> *breath, and the other well-known signs of the disease.*
> *During the sixth day there occurs a great diminution*
> *of the contractile force of the heart and voluntary*
> *muscles, the pulse becomes very feeble and thready, the*
> *respiratory movements are modified, and the animal*
> *sometimes shows such weakness in the limbs that it has*
> *even been thought that some special paralytic affection*
> *of the spinal nerve must exist. The temperature now*
> *rapidly falls, and signs of a great diminution in the*
> *normal chemical changes in the body appear.*[5]

Cattle usually die by the sixth day.

Since the fall of Kiev, rinderpest has been a rolling horror for Europe's bovines, with outbreaks periodically annihilating herds across the continent. It struck England in 1348–1349, when the human population was still reeling from the Black Death. The herdsmen, dead or frightened of returning to the blighted pastures, let their cattle roam free, spreading the plague across the countryside. From 1480 to 1481, Germany and Switzerland lost an entire third of their cattle to the disease. In the nineteenth century, it struck Napoleon's baggage animals during his invasion of Russia, a disaster that likely helped convince him to turn tail for Paris. But as bad as these historical outbreaks certainly were, no one imagined the scale of the catastrophe that lay ahead.

The Hull Docks, Northern England, 1865, and newspapers were full of railway stories. British investors had been particularly attentive to accounts of new tracks stitching the mines and farms of eastern Europe together with the factories of the West. Commodities like lumber and ore rolled in bulk toward the sunset, and the industrial towns belched out textiles and steamships in return. Notwithstanding Robert Bakewell's innovations in stock breeding, factory workers needed more food, and domestic producers couldn't keep up with the demand for beef and milk. Russian cattle were cheap, and now they were available for import. Entrepreneurs who bought them in Minsk and sold them in London stood to make a lucrative bundle of sterling.

But not if a prickly scientist named John Gamgee had any say in the matter. A veterinarian by training (before veterinary medicine was an established profession), and an iconoclast by temper, Gamgee understood that if diseased cattle moved from farm to farm, so did the disease. And if that disease were rinderpest, there would be no more farms from which to move. He wrote vociferous letters to Parliament, demanding controls on the movement of animals, and immediate slaughter and quarantine at the first flare of infection. Nobody listened to him, though. The opportunity for profiteering in beef was simply too ripe.

The man who opened Pandora's box was a cattle trader named John Burchell. His specialty was buying inexpensive eastern European cows, shipping them across the Baltic, and selling them to English butchers and dairies. Burchell had qualms about importing sick beasts—he insisted that he had once resisted pressure from the Prussian government to buy diseased stock. But his compunctions didn't extend to seemingly healthy cows that had merely been pastured alongside sick ones. In Estonia, he loaded such a cargo onto the S.S. *Tonning* and, knowing that the port of Hull on Britain's east coast was notorious for its lax inspections standards, he delivered a shipload of percolating rinderpest into northern England.[6]

These animals were no thoroughbreds. Eastern European cattle, though known for their hardiness, came in every size, color, and measure of quality. They had traveled for two days by train to reach their port of departure, never being cleaned, perhaps never being watered. Then it was another eight days of airless enclosure in the hold of the *Tonning* before being entrained, again, in Hull.

Once in Hull, two veterinarians signed off on the shipment to mark it "clean" (one of them later confessed to negligence). In late May 1865, the animals embarked on a train, and, twenty-four hours later, were being auctioned off at London's cattle market. Within days, they had mixed with herds in every corner of Britain.

Cows throughout Britain began to die, first sporadically, then in droves. Within six months, six thousand fresh infections were being reported per week. Before the disease ebbed, a total of 420,000 animals perished, and it would take British farmers a quarter century to rebuild their stock. The situation was just as bad on the Continent. The rinderpest pandemic of 1865 is estimated to have killed two hundred million cattle across Europe.[7]

John Gamgee watched the deaths, appalled. At the time, the "foul vapors" theory of contagion was generally accepted, and many of the farmers and cattle traders of the day believed that disease spontaneously blossomed in different geographical areas. But Gamgee was convinced that this was nonsense. He believed that healthy animals became infected by coming into contact with sick ones. Sanitation was also a factor, and he held railroad cars and ships' holds in particular contempt. Writing in 1863 he describes diseased animals left: "lying thick on the bottom of the trucks . . . , charged with poison which readily infects any animals coming in contact with it"[8]

Gamgee was a devotee of this new "germ theory," a radical idea that had yet to infect the public imagination. It would be another decade before Robert Koch proved that anthrax was caused by the bacterium *Bacillus anthrasis*, and fifteen years before Louis Pasteur developed a cholera vaccine. At the beginning of the 1865 outbreak, however, most people had little concept of germs. They thought that applying veterinary science to the problem of rinderpest would prove more expensive than the disease itself.[9] For example, in 1864, Gamgee had successfully lobbied Parliament to bring forward two bills that would have given veterinarians power to curtail the import and export of livestock. Both were defeated in the name of economic freedom. And, a year later, Burchell brought his cows to England.

The response to the 1865 outbreak was a tragedy of errors. First, Parliament authorized the appointment of official veterinarians in regions affected by rinderpest. The appointments were derailed by politics and corruption, as well as the fact that few people had any qualifications to practice animal medicine. Worse, however, was the behavior of butchers. As soon as a cow showed any symptoms, butchers would slaughter the animal and sell its meat before anyone noticed that it had been dripping contagion. The rotten carcasses were shipped around the country. And so was the rinderpest.

The government's second response was to appoint a Royal Commission to study the disease. Its second report, tabled in November of 1865, recommended restrictions on the transport of livestock but did not recommend the immediate slaughter of diseased animals. All the while, Gamgee tried to drum up support for stauncher measures, measures he knew would work, but measures that were difficult for politicians to swallow. These were to slaughter, to quarantine, and to cease transport of livestock.

The Royal Commission tabled a third report in early in 1866, by which time the epidemic had stripped England's meadows of their cows. Faced with the ruin of an industry, the report grudgingly admitted: "The way in which the disease broke out . . . [is] conclusive evidence against the assumption of an occult atmospheric condition, and in favour of its spread by multiplication in the bodies of living animals."[10] Germ theory had, too late, won over public opinion.

Of course, the only solution to the immediate problem was the poleax and a halt to importation. But by 1866, the damage was irre-

versible. It shouldn't have been so disastrous—there had been prece-
dents for quarantine as far back as the seventeenth century, when a
doctor named Bernardino Ramazzini wrote the first concise guide on
the benefits of containing animal diseases. In the eighteenth century,
Pope Clement XI's personal physician, one Giovianni Lancisi, urged
his employer to order diseased cattle be slaughtered and buried, and
markets closed at the first sign of an outbreak. Legend has it that any
churchman caught disobeying these edicts would have been imprisoned for life, while laypeople were hanged, drawn, and quartered. In
England in 1714, Thomas Bates, the royal surgeon to King George I,
proposed a similar set of safeguards (without the hanging and mutilation) and eradicated an outbreak within a matter of months.

But these were momentary flashes of caution. The customary response to disease was useless panic.

In 1841, a shipload of Russian cattle arrived in Egypt's port of Alex-
andria. Until then, Africa had been spared the blight of rinderpest, but
within a few months of this particular delivery, 665,000 African cows
had died of the disease. One Lady Duff Gordon, writing from Alexan-
dria, complained about the complete disappearance of milk from the
marketplace. Despite the loss of these animals, the disease had burned
itself out and Africa remained free of rinderpest, for a time.

A second outbreak, forty years later, was much more calamitous,
even by the calamitous standards of Africa.[11] This one was sparked by
animals imported by Italian soldiers disembarking at the port city of
Massawa in Eritrea in 1885. Rinderpest tore through East Africa destroying the fabric of daily life. A local nun wrote "the people, having
nothing more to eat, . . . boil the skin of cattle destroyed by the epidemic." An American envoy estimated that 92 percent of East Africa's
cattle were dead by 1890.

Since the disease coincided with a drought, herds were congregated around the few damp waterholes that remained. Intimacy spread the infection. An Ethiopian named Alaqa Lamma wrote that only one of his father's three hundred cattle survived the plague. On a journey to Addis Ababa, Lamma observed a landscape stripped of animal life: in a town called Salaleheé he only saw a single calf; crossing the mountains he counted a mere six oxen.[12]

By 1896, rinderpest had appeared south of the Zambezi River, the natural dividing line that had isolated southern Africa from northerly infections, and by the spring of 1897, it had ravaged South African herds. Since Africans relied on ox-drawn carts for trade and communication, the roads became disease corridors. Soon, the deaths meant that villages could no longer plow their fields or carry grain to market. They had no milk and no means to travel. Since cattle comprised most of Africa's wealth, the plague destroyed the equivalent of a continent's savings accounts. French missionary Fracois Coillard described the scene in 1897:

> *[Rinderpest] mowed down the whole bovine race in*
> *its passage. Hundreds of carcasses lay here and there,*
> *on the road side or piled up in the fields. . . . the carrion*
> *lay there, putrefying everywhere. More than nine*
> *hundred wagons, loaded with merchandise, without*
> *teams or drivers, stood abandoned along the . . .*
> *road. Never in the memory of man has such a thing*
> *been seen.*[13]

Rinderpest's virulence was savage enough to bring down herds of buffalo and bison. Giraffes went blind. Oryx, elands, and the greater kudu all died en masse. And as the wild grazers perished, so did the big cats that ate them. With the game animals gone and the predators starving, trees began to creep into the savannah. It was at the end of the nineteenth century that most of East Africa's forests emerged.[14] Landscapes like the Masai Mara—where today it's hard to throw a

stone without hitting a gazelle and an attendant van of rapt photogra-
phers—were desolate. One observer commented that a visitor could
"wander . . . without seeing any more wildlife than in two hours at the
Berlin zoo."[15]

In 1920, a shipload of Indian zebu cows arrived in Antwerp via Brazil,
bringing rinderpest with them. This Belgian outbreak was the final straw.
In 1924, governments established the World Organization for Animal
Health to eradicate the disease.[16] This, along with vaccination programs,
the immediate slaughter of infected animals, and controls on movement,
prevented rinderpest from taking hold in the Americas, Australia, and
New Zealand. Africa was, as always, another story.

As well as spreading continental ruin and desolation, rinderpest
had far-reaching consequences for science. It spurred the acceptance of
germ theory and the establishment of veterinary medicine. John Gamgee's work on infected cows was especially useful in these regards—his
clinical studies were the first to use thermometers to measure fevers in
sick patients. Gamgee took his Cassandra prophecies to the United
States, where he embarked on a new line of research into refrigeration.
His advice on disease control, still sound despite being 150 years old,
shares a practical fate with that of flossing—everyone knows it's right,
but it's often honored in the breach.

Today's international cattle and beef trade is immense, shuttling
countless head of cattle between continents and accounting for hundreds of billions in annual revenues.[17] Rinderpest isn't as murderous
as in the past and has, with difficulty, been eradicated from many
parts of the world. But recurring outbreaks of hoof-and-mouth disease and mad cow disease (not to mention the evergreen paranoia of
avian flu) keep the greasy charnel fires burning on both sides of the
Atlantic.

During rinderpest's heyday, a Victorian clergyman called John
Mason Neale published a poem in the Manchester Guardian newspaper. Titled "Hymn to the Cattle Plague," the poem urged Neale's readers to reflect on the human agency of the disaster:

So pity them [the cows] thy guiltless creature
Who not less man's suffering share
For our sins it is they perish
Let them profit by our prayer.

The cows didn't profit much from prayer. What they really needed in order to replenish their numbers was a French chemist named Louis Pasteur.

◆ Chemical Solutions ◆
Making Food Last Longer

In the years when the British navy was the scourge of Napoleon and the shield of empire, patriotic English landlords decided it was in the best interests of the king and country to shoot acorns out of cannons. This was history's weirdest act of reforestation, a literal attempt to blast the next generation of fighting ships into the hillside. Less violent forestry didn't work much better. Today, the United Kingdom is largely treeless. The Yorkshire Dales are typical. Odd coppices of oaks and a few dying twentieth-century pine plantations are the only breaks in a quilt of stone walls and pasture.[18] This is old dairy country, a landscape built for cattle.

The Dale valleys are tame, habitable, and seemingly concocted by Victorian novelists. They're crisscrossed with country lanes that sport "wild roses in summer . . . nuts and blackberries in autumn . . . but whose best winter delight lay in its utter solitude and leafless repose" (Charlotte Brontë, *Jane Eyre*, chapter 12). If the valleys are Charlotte Brontë, the hilltops belong to her sister Emily. These are a palette of heather, scrag, and black winds—savage Heathcliff instead of mildly Byronic Mr. Rochester. The lower slopes are a pale, green checkerboard of pasture laboriously picked clean of stones—hence the endless, stacked walls.

ༀⓒ

CULINARY INTERLUDE

Roast Beef and Yorkshire Pudding

Instead of ridicule and cruel jokes about spotted dick, English cuisine nowadays elicits curiosity and even pleasant surprise. One of the long-neglected pillars of British eating is the pudding—a more or less meaningless term that embraces foods as disparate as pies and varieties of sausage. The Yorkshire Pud is the most famous and, when served with a slab of roast and gravy, is the basis of a traditional Yorkshire Sunday dinner. This recipe comes from Muriel Appleyard, grandmother of one of the authors.

Roast a sirloin or standing rib according to any recipe preferred, making sure to throw in a few potatoes and parsnips. For the pudding, beat one egg, ¾ cup of milk, and ¼ cup of water. Sift together 1 cup of flour, 1 teaspoon of tartar, ½ teaspoon soda, ½ teaspoon salt. Add this to the milk and egg mixture to make a batter and add a tablespoon of melted butter. Then pour 1 tablespoon hot drippings from the roast into each depression of a muffin tin and place the tin in an oven heated to 400 degrees. When the grease begins to smoke, add a dollop of batter to each muffin receptacle and bake for twenty minutes. The pudding should rise into a crisp, hollow puff. Serve alongside roast beef slathered with gravy and vegetables.

In many of the dales, at intervals of about a half kilometer, stand field barns. Built entirely out of stone with slate roofs, these abandoned structures are two stories high and no more than ten meters long, often melding into hillsides so that hay could be forked through the upper windows without the necessity of ladders. The barns used to be winter homes for cows. Today's giant Frisians wouldn't have fit inside, but a hundred and fifty years ago, four or five little gray-brown shorthorns

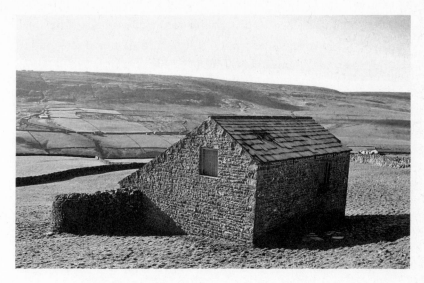

NINETEENTH-CENTURY DAIRY BARN IN THE YORKSHIRE DALES, UK.
Credit: Photo by Evan Fraser.

would have passed the snowy months in safety, tethered in their flag-
stone stalls, only emerging for a daily turn in the paved yard in front of
the door.

In the summer, these cows pulled plows and carts. Once winter set
in, their energies were devoted solely toward milking, to which they
submitted once per day, twice in the case of a prodigy. Farmers collected their manure for the pastures. They helped mine lead and clear
land for new fields. Unlike American pioneers, who had merely to con-
tend with forests, Yorkshire farmers were shifting acres of great boul-
ders, dropped by the vanishing glaciers of the last Ice Age. Clearing a
few dozen meters took a generation.

This was hard land, and it made for hard people and animals. It
also made for a spectacular view. Writing in the early twentieth century, country veterinarian James Herriot described "a wild panorama
of tumbling fells [that] . . . rolled away and lost itself in the crimson
and gold ribbons of the western sky."[19] Far from being moist emerald
hillocks, however, these dairy lands of a hundred and fifty years ago
were flinty and sharp. They were also isolated. Before the nineteenth

century, no one needed to bring milk very far to market. The small herds would have kept the nearest village and manor in cream, but their product would never have traveled. Milk is designed to be drunk at the moment of expression. Left in air, it quickly goes bad. If milk is kept clean, it will simply spoil, fermenting with bacteria that turn its sugars into lactic acid. Under unsanitary conditions it is lethal, an ideal broth for tuberculosis, salmonella, and *E. coli*. So throughout history, it's been imperative that milk drinkers stay within a day's journey of the nearest lactating cow. Small, local dairy farms have always been the only means of delivering fresh milk to thirsty customers. Large, centralized herds, like the ones that emerged in the beef industry, would have gone to waste.

Unlike water, milk can't be sterilized by simple boiling. Overheating causes proteins (called micelles) to glom together and curdle. Before the nineteenth century, then, the only way to store milk for any length of time was to curdle it—hence the popularity of cheese, yogurt, and butter. Butter, for example, is made when the membranes between butterfat globules are broken apart through slow churning. While whole, particles slip around one another. The broken ones, however, squish together and clump. Because slightly soured milk still makes good butter, milk could be collected for a couple of days before undergoing churning. Butter is compact, dense, and has a small surface area compared to liquid, so it takes a long time to spoil, and the addition of salt kills some of the more opportunistic bacteria that might be tempted to lodge in it. It was a good use for milk that would otherwise have been dumped.

And then, in 1862, millennia of assumptions evaporated. A chemist named Louis Pasteur had been conducting early experiments with germs, demonstrating, for instance, that boiled broth kept out of the open air didn't grow mold, while free-breathing broth turned furry. He concluded that mold must be made by agents in the air. Building on this, he worked out a method of slow-heating liquids to a temperature just shy of a boil. The process reduced bacteria without killing everything in the way of texture and taste, a discovery that radically lengthened a liquid's storage life. Pasteur didn't apply his method to milk, as he was more interested in wine (milk got its treatment from a Czech chemist named Franz Ritter von Soxhlet). But by the late 1800s, milk had gained a longevity of weeks if stored in cool conditions.

If fresh milk was no longer the mayfly of the dairy world, then there was no reason that it couldn't be produced in bulk, and then stored, transported, and sold to urbanites far from the countryside. Under these conditions, small local dairy farms couldn't hope to produce enough milk to service the city markets (although most of the giant milk producers active today are twentieth-century firms that branched into fresh milk from related avenues: Parmalat started as a pasteurization plant, Land o' Lakes as a butter cooperative, and Dean was a condensed milk cannery). Whereas shelf life had once kept production low, now the only limit was the vibrancy of the udder. The economies of scale for dairies exploded with pasteurization and dairies bought each other up or went out of business and, shorn of their cattle's cropping lips, the hillsides of places like Switzerland and Yorkshire and Massachusetts began to sink into thorny desolation. In Yorkshire, sheep replaced cows on the hilltops. Instead of turning scrub into milk, dairy cows now congregated into much larger herds that grazed richer pastures—land that would once have been fenced for tillage.

Once farmers knew they could sell as much milk as they could produce, they, like their compatriots in beef, began to breed their cattle with an eye toward gigantism. In the Dales, farmers purged their herds of the stout little shorthorns that had grazed the hills for centuries. They wanted honey-coated Jerseys, fawn Guernseys, tough Brown Swiss, and red Scottish Ayrshires—the world's champion milkers.

The most notable international success was the Dutch Holstein, the most famous of all cows for its black-and-white spotted coat, its bulging udders, and its granite placidity. In the United States, a New Englander named Winthrop Chenery imported the first Holstein cow from the Netherlands in 1852, and these monochromatic marvels came to dominate the milking business in both North America and Europe. Today, the American Holstein herd accounts for approximately nine million animals that each produces about ten thousand kilograms of milk per annum.[20] Dairy cows are vastly outnumbered by the approximately one hundred million American beeves, but they could still float a reasonably sized battleship on their multiple daily excretions.

Holsteins, having one of the largest gene pools of any cattle breed, have found themselves at the forefront of bovine breeding and cloning. In 2000, Canadian veterinary scientists used cells from an exceptionally virile Holstein bull named Hanoverhill Starbuck to hatch a healthy male calf.[21] It was history's first prize bull clone. Starbuck kept an extremely full calendar and produced quite a few conventional, artificially inseminated offspring: he sold 685,000 doses of his semen to herds in forty-five countries, breeding more than two hundred thousand milk-rich daughters.[22]

At the same time as Holsteins were starting to overflow the milk pails of New England, the desolation brought about by the American Civil War in the South was creating a new landscape, a new economy, and a strange new breed of cow. At its peak, this animal would number in the tens of millions, but it would also prove to be something less than the sum of its ancestry. The modern American beef cow was about to be born.

♦ Cowboys *and* Barbed Wire ♦

The American Civil War was ancient violence inflicted on an industrial scale.[23] It revived old horrors, like massed infantry armed with muskets, pikes, and sabers, but it quickened them with telegraph lines and railways, and mowed them down with bullets spat from machines. Bloodshed was, for the first time, tinted with gear oil. As went the war, so went the country. By 1865, the United States ceased to be a land of homespun rural stereotypes and emerged as a modern nation—less whitewashed farmhouse than brick chimney and tenement. Many things passed away in the Civil War. Not least was the hoary old role of cattle as jack-of-all-animals.

When the western states and territories lost their young men to the regiments, there was no one left to round up the cattle. Nor did the remaining ranchers have enough hands to drive the stock across hundreds of miles to market. So the cows wandered free. These weren't Bakewell's overbred beeves or easygoing Holsteins. American beef cows had yet to be "improved" and the cattle of the Civil War were longhorns, descended from the rangy Spanish cows brought over by de Guzmán and his fellow conquistadors. They were an anachronism. Having crossed into Texas from Mexico over a period of hundreds of years, they had learned to ford the quick rivers, hunch their shoulders against the heat, and survive by cropping pale prairie grass. They weren't especially beefy, but they were good at resisting hard weather and rattlesnakes. They likely had some *Bos indicus* blood, which kept them from broiling in the sunlight, but they didn't have the shoulder hump common to zebus today. Their coats were solid reds and browns, although some sported a blue-black sheen, or dapples of dirty white.

The original Spanish name for the animal was *criollo*—a word commonly used for mixed-race people—but by 1865, English speakers called them Texas longhorns. The longhorn was a useless milker and had inherited the truculence of its Spanish forefathers, but it thrived on neglect, ate anything that sported even a trace of chlorophyll, and had a knack for easy pregnancies.[24] In this, and in horn and body shape, it took after its ancestor, the *Bos primigenius,* the aurochs.[25] Steers frequently reached a horn span of six feet from tip to tip, and there are records of eight-and-a-half-foot spans.[26] More importantly, the longhorn was impervious to bovine babesiosis, a tickborne disease also known as Texas fever or the bloody murrain.[27] Expensive imports like the Holstein or Aberdeen Angus died in a matter of days after infection, but a diseased longhorn trundled on. As carriers, however, they spread the parasite to the soft, European immigrants, snuffing attempts to introduce new breeds to the West.

Longhorn ranching was a hodgepodge, like the animals themselves. Ranchers burned pasture at the end of the summer, both to fertilize new shoots and to torch the legions of ticks and other bloodsuckers native to the countryside. In the spring, mounted ranch-hands rode into the winter forage lands and herded the cows, branding the new-born calves, and selecting their pick for market. The ones not tagged for slaughter returned to the wild for another season of freedom. It was a system descended from the Spanish ranches in Andalusia, with strains of the Celtic-British from the west of England.[28] The use of lassos, for example, was Iberian. Dogs and whips, commonly employed in Florida ranches, were English.[29]

Longhorns had an obnoxious habit of bolting at the first glimpse of a human being and getting stuck in thickets, gullies, and other inaccessible places. The men who dragged and herded them back into the range were necessarily rugged, persistent, and sunburned. They became a symbol of the American "can-do" spirit, but the word *cowboy* wasn't always so patriotically charged. The first "cowboys" were actually Loyalist marauders wreaking havoc in the hinterland around New York during the War of Independence. Most of the genre's tropes—the six-shooters, the quick-draw dueling—are later exaggerations by serial writers, and it's unlikely that bison-eating Native Americans ever engaged in much rustling. Like the longhorn, the cowboy was a mixed creature.

It's hard to exaggerate the cowboy's immensity as an icon and pop cultural motif. A lone rider, unmistakably crowned, against a vista of tumbleweeds and jutting plateaux is the hero of an American myth of individualism, laconic valor, and a steady hand on the trigger. It's a myth shaped by movies, with John Wayne as its cardinal reenactor. Joan Didion writes:

> . . . *when John Wayne rode through my childhood,*
> *and perhaps through yours, he determined forever*
> *the shape of certain of our dreams. . . . And in a world*
> *we understood early to be characterized by venality*
> *and doubt and paralyzing ambiguities, he suggested*
> *another world, one which may or may not have existed*
> *ever but in any case existed no more: a place where a*

*man could move free, could make his own code and
live by it; a world in which, if a man did what he had
to do, he could one day take the girl and go riding
through the draw and find himself home free, not in
a hospital with something wrong inside, not in a high
bed with the flowers and the drugs and the forced
smiles, but there at the bend in the bright river, the
cottonwoods shimmering in the early morning sun.[30]*

In the twentieth century, movies showed cowboy life as an idyll of open skies, lungfuls of prairie air and cheroots, and freedom to shoot varmints. Cowboys even assumed a tag of chivalry. Gene Autry, Hollywood's most popular singing cowboy, sang ballads about honest cowpokes who never shot first and who helped ladies in distress, respected the flag, and wore clean white hats.[31] Add chain mail, and it's not much of a jump to Amadis of Gaul.

The historical cowboy, not his dime-store shadow, was closer in spirit to Cuchulainn and his wild raiders than to a moony knight errant. An anonymous Englishman who worked the Texas drives of the 1880s describes his fellow cowboys' "primitive code of honor" as including "honesty, courage, sensitive pride, stoic indifference to pain, and, above all, a violent vengefulness against insult."[32] He may as well have been talking about the court of King Conchobor, or of the Masai. The Hollywood legend did, however, get two points right: there was once an open range in the United States, and the cows walked a very, very long way to market.

Clichés don't spring unbidden from the heads of writers—they need a seed. In the case of cowboys, one of these seeds was the career of Charles Goodnight, cowboy extraordinaire. The son of poor "dirt" farmers in 1836 in Macoupin County, Illinois, Goodnight was five years old when his father died of pneumonia, and eleven when his mother remarried and moved the family to Texas.[33] Stories claim that Goodnight rode bareback during the eight-hundred-mile journey, straddling a white-faced mare named Blaze.

Abandoning the schoolroom after six unprofitable months, Good-night's education was in the heroic style; he learned hunting and track-ing at the knee of an Indian mentor, and as a young man, he worked on an oxen train, supervised a crew of slaves, and tried his hand at ranching. In the 1850s, he worked driving cattle to Colorado to sell to hungry prospectors. Later, he signed up as a guide during the Indian Wars, volunteering to lead federal troops to Native campsites. His most famous engagement occurred on December 18, 1860, when he rode with a detachment of soldiers to a Comanche camp where, after the gunfire died down and the bodies had been cleared, they discovered Cynthia Ann Parker, a white captive who became nationally famous for having married a brave with whom she raised a family of Coman-che children.

Goodnight fought on the side of the Confederates during the Civil War, and when his term of service expired in 1864, he aban-doned the cause and returned home. Upon arrival in Texas, he was delighted to find that his cattle had kept themselves occupied in strenuous procreation. So had all the other longhorns in Texas. Herds that had numbered a few dozen head before the war now amounted to hundreds. Herds that had numbered hundreds had bred them-selves into the thousands. Far from suffering from neglect, the semi-feral longhorns delighted in being left alone while their owners butchered one another—in 1866, Texas cattle numbered five million head.[34]

Even better, since all the ranch-hands had enlisted, the herds had mingled. No one had been around to swing a branding iron. Now, an enterprising rancher with a horse and lasso could round up and claim as many animals as he could catch. But since so many cows suddenly appeared on the market, they weren't worth much. Goodnight and an old friend named Oliver Loving realized that army outposts in New Mexico had no access to the glut. They would pay top government dol-lars for beef. Smelling an opportunity, the two entrepreneurs drove their herd southwest to Horsehead Crossing on the Pecos River, then north to Fort Sumner. It was a long drive, but it made a splendid profit. They did it again. And then again, dubbing their venture the Goodnight-Loving Train, the route of which became one of the most heavily trodden roads in Texas. It wasn't an easy one to walk. The weather was hard and the Natives resentful. Loving died in a gun battle with Indians in 1867.

Despite the violent loss of his friend and business partner, the early death of his father, a childhood of poverty, and fighting on the losing side of the Civil War, Goodnight could consider himself a lucky man. Britain—and much of Europe—had just lost innumerable cattle to the plague that Gamgee had fought.[35] The horror of the Irish potato famine had finally convinced the English government to allow food to be imported. Europe wanted beef. And so did the United States. After the Civil War, cities like New York and Chicago mushroomed with millions of immigrants from the countryside and abroad. These urban markets paid up to $50 per head, easily ten times the cost of a steer in Texas. Surging demand coincided with the final defeat of the Indians, five years after the Battle of Little Big Horn in 1876, and endless seas of grass opened up for grazing in Colorado, Wyoming, Montana, Idaho, and the Dakotas. Texas, which produced an apparently unlimited supply of calves, was the logical source to stock the prairies.[36]

Goodnight thought carefully about how to exploit the situation. His experience in long-range drives had taught him that cowboys at the end of a drive were at the mercy of local buyers. Their animals, having hoofed through the dust for thousands of miles, arrived at the market skinny and underfed. The cowboys themselves weren't much better off—they were exhausted and desperate to collect their money for the journey home. What they needed, Goodnight realized, was a lush pasture adjacent to the market town, a place where man and beast could refresh their strength, girth, and composure. To this end, he secured grazing rights for his cattle at the ends of his drives. If beef prices had fallen when the cows arrived, the animals could wait in comfort for a more favorable moment before going to auction.

Beginning in 1866, the "long drives" of Western legend lasted for about twenty-five years, moving an estimated 5.4 million animals to urban markets along routes like the Chisholm Trail, linking southern Texas with Abilene, Kansas, and the railroad to Chicago. The ranchers made millions on the backs of the longhorns. Goodnight, due to his fattened steers, became one of the wealthiest men in America. But, like every economic fairy tale, it ended not happily ever after, but with a humbling moral.

In 1885, 350,000 cattle made the long drives east. In 1886, the number was virtually zero. Money, technology, and disease had killed the system.

During the boom years in longhorn beef, the profit on raising a calf to slaughter amounted to 400–700 percent. Foreign investors, particularly the British, read the figures with dry lips and quaking fingers. In 1879, the Anglo-American Cattle Company, Ltd. was incorporated with capital of $350,000, which it used to buy up dozens of ranches and twenty-seven thousand head of cattle. Other investors followed its example, and by 1882 there were nine international companies operating in America's cattle lands.

Nor was it merely the London financier who saw riches in a cowpat. Immigrants from the East flooded into the Great Plains, convinced that fortune lay over the next hump of prairie grass. Between 1870 and 1890 the Dakotas swelled from a population of 14,000 to 719,000. Nebraska, Kansas, and Texas were no different. Timber frames replaced the old sod houses. Plows tore up the pasture. An early twentieth-century chronicler wrote:

> Into a region of long-horned steers, hard riding men,
> boots, spurs, branding irons, saddles, ropes, and six
> shooters, [the new arrivals] brought plows and hoes,
> pitchforks, churns, cook stoves, rocking chairs, feather
> beds, pillows, dogs, cats, pigs, and chickens, but most
> important of all, wives and children. To a region of
> sour dough bread, beef steak, bacon, dried apples,

beans, flapjacks, and coffee were brought salt rising
bread, buttermilk biscuits, pies, cakes, doughnuts,
preserves, jellies, custards, and fresh vegetables.[37]

This was an invasion, a cultural shift from a feudal world of un-couth mounted warriors and open pasture to a modern scene of small farms, schoolrooms, and Victorian social norms.[38] It wasn't long before the new arrivals began to talk of progress. An immediate candidate for improvement was the source of all the riches and ambition, the long-horn cow. It was stringy. It was thin. Wouldn't a pure European beef cow prove superior?

The answer, at first, was no, because it would be dead from Texas fever. But Pasteur's germ theory had begun to percolate among the ranchers, and investigators discovered that the longhorn was not only a survivor of the disease, but also a carrier. Even old John Gamgee, scourge of rinderpest, arrived in the Wild West to pronounce a recom-mendation of strict quarantine laws on longhorns.[39]

The new breed of farmers read the newspaper reports, and they didn't like the idea of infected longhorns traipsing through their fresh-painted fences. They wanted to outlaw the long drives. One nineteenth-century rancher is recorded wondering how the government could continue to allow the drives that left "the germs of disease . . ." given that this had already cost "hundreds of thousand of dollars from losses incurred without any compensation or direct benefit."[40]

Public opinion shifted. Even Kansans, who had once viewed the long drives as an opportunity to sell things to Texans, turned against their old business partners. One Kansan stated that as soon as the Texas herds set hoof on private property, the smart farmer "coolly loads his gun, and joins his neighbors. They mean to kill, do kill, and will keep killing until the drove takes the back track."[41]

Vigilante cow-shooting came to be known as the "Winchester Quarantine."[42] It wasn't unjustified. In the mid-1880s, Texas fever in-fected 19,229 head of Kansas cattle, killing 2,300. Two counties alone lost more than 2,000. Small farmers couldn't survive such a financial blow, and losses from the outbreak topped $75,400.[43] Bowing to the inevitable, in 1867 the Kansas legislature established a "dead line" that ran across the southern part of the state, making it illegal to drive Texas cattle north and east of the demarcation. Another outbreak in 1884 cost the state $500,000, and by 1885 the dead line had crept so far north that the entire state was quarantined.[44]

The quarantine didn't work, at least not at first. Cowboys have a reputation for ignoring inconvenient laws, and no number of petulant farmers can stop a herd of three thousand determined longhorns. It took barbed wire to do that.

At about the same time as Goodnight was stocking his herds and forging his trails, one Joseph F. Glidden of Dekalb, Illinois, was strolling through a county fair when, by chance, he saw a wooden rail studded with nails hanging on a smooth wire fence. Inspired by the image, he went home and used a coffee grinder to cut some metal barbs which he placed at intervals along a length of smooth wire, securing them with a second length of wire twisted around the first.[45] It was a simple contraption, and it was revolutionary. With it, farmers could fence huge areas of land without the high cost of timber or stone. They could separate their herds from those of their neighbors without fear of mingling. Most of all, they could stake private claims on grazing land, quickly fencing it off from neighbors and, worse, itinerant herds.[46] If changing demographics weakened the long drive, barbed wire strangled it.

By the 1880s, "the devil's rope" hung across the pastures at river fords and watering holes, its metal spools unfurled by small landowners who hated the annual depredations inflicted by the longhorns. There was nothing drovers like Goodnight could do. Nothing, not even the stubborn will of the longhorns, could disentangle the trails. When the railway arrived—reaching Dallas in 1873 and spinning outward like a spider's web—it gobbled up the Chicago trade, and when refrigerated cars first rolled in 1875, it was a foolish rancher who didn't realize that the future was iron and steam.

The longhorn, like the cowboy, didn't survive the end of the century. Meatier animals like the Aberdeen Angus took its place, while the last cowboys drifted into "Wild West Shows," before vanishing utterly into the burgeoning cities, like all the other rootless spirits of America.

ᔫᐪ

CULINARY INTERLUDE

Barbecue and Beef Jerky

Southern barbecue has its origins on the plantations, where slaves cooked cheap pork cuts like shoulders and ribs by slow-grilling them in earthen pits. Texas beef barbecue is also pit-cooked, although today the pit takes the form of a stainless steel smoker with a Teflon grate. Murderous controversy surrounds nearly every aspect of barbecuing. Marinade or rub? Trim the fat or leave it on? Sauce or dry? But it's generally agreed that the key ingredients are smoke and time.

Texas barbecued brisket recipes are easy to come by, but since most ordinary citizens lack a smoker, they're not terribly advantageous. This one, from the Texas Beef Council, merely requires use of a large grill and ten hours of leisure.

Mix ¼ cup salt with ¼ cup brown sugar, ¼ cup white sugar, ¼ cup cumin, ¼ cup chili powder, ¼ cup black pepper, ½ cup paprika, and 2 tablespoons cayenne pepper. Rub onto a 10-pound brisket. Build a mesquite fire on one side of a grill and place the meat on the opposite side, so none of it is above the flames. Close the grill cover and open the vent a crack. Stoke the fire when necessary, keeping the temperature at about 170° Fahrenheit, and cook for about ten hours. Slice it thin, against the grain.[47] Barbecued brisket is among the world's most pliant meats—it's as soft and moist as an oiled sponge—but smoke gives it personality.

On the opposite end of the cowboy dining spectrum is dry, wooden jerky, a camp food that's lately surged in popularity as a snacking alternative to fried corn or potatoes. The word *jerky* derives from the Peruvian *charqui* meaning "dried meat."[48] Most cultures throughout history have cut meat into strips and preserved it by drying, either through salting or simply hanging it in the sun.[49] According to the North Dakota State

University College of Agriculture, Food Systems and Natural Resources, the process can be duplicated at home without much risk of poisoning.

Slice 5 pounds of lean beef along the grain and sprinkle with 3 tablespoons salt, 2 tablespoons ground pepper, and 2 tablespoons sugar. Refrigerate for twenty-four hours, then pound the meat on both sides before dipping into a bath of liquid smoke for one to two seconds. Dissolve ½ cup salt, ½ cup sugar, and 2 tablespoons black pepper in a gallon of water to make brine, bringing to a low boil. Immerse the strips in the liquid until they turn gray, then lay them on the clean top rack of an oven. Leave the door of the oven ajar and cook at 120–150 degrees for between nine and twenty-four hours. The meat is done if it cracks when bent, but doesn't break.[50]

◆   Bubbly Creek *and the* Union Stock Yards   ◆

As the Civil War ground to a halt in 1864, a consortium of Chicago investors decided that the future was in meat. Guessing that a peaceful country would have an enormous appetite, they bought a large swamp in the southwest part of the city and turned it into America's biggest centralized stockyard, laying in waterways, railway tracks, and processing plants. It opened for business on Christmas Day 1865. By 1900, it filled 475 acres. Of the millions of Texan beeves sent east in the late nineteenth century, a majority of them died here. The waste from the carcasses was so torrential, and so rancid, that the part of the Chicago River into which it flowed earned the nickname "Bubbly Creek."[51]

The Union Stock Yards, as they were known, produced 82 percent of America's meat at the turn of the century. Never had the world known such commonplace plenty—canned beef, canned sausages, and cooking lard by the pound. The price for cheap meat was a workplace environment out of the mind of Hieronymous Bosch. Upton Sinclair described the horrors in his 1906 book *The Jungle,* in which he showed how the factories treated immigrant workers and their families much like the animals that they carved and boiled. This description of the

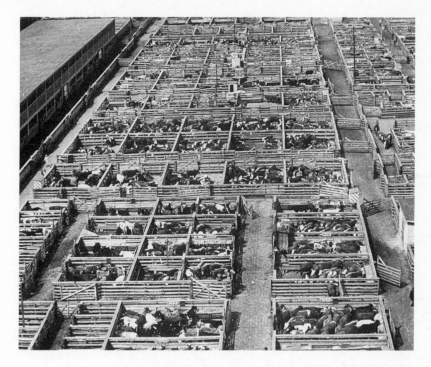

CATTLE PROCESSING AT THE OMAHA, NEBRASKA, STOCK
YARD IN THE 1950s, WHICH WAS SECOND IN SIZE ONLY
TO THE CHICAGO STOCK YARD. *Credit: Photo by Bernard
Hoffman/Time Life Pictures/Getty Images.*

killing floor comes just after a boy working the lard machine has his
ears frozen and literally rubbed off:

> On the killing beds you were apt to be covered in blood,
> and it would freeze solid; if you leaned against a pillar,
> you would freeze to that. . . . The men would tie up
> their feet in newspapers and old sacks, and these would
> be soaked in blood and frozen, and then soaked again,
> and so on, until by nighttime a man would be walking
> on great lumps the size of the feet of an elephant.
> Now and then, when the bosses were not looking, you
> would see them plunging their feet and ankles into the
> steaming hot carcass of the steer.[52]

As a portrait of industrial barbarism, *The Jungle* still has the power
to shock. This famous passage caused swoons in genteel parlors across
the country:

> There were those who made the tins for the canned
> meat; and their hands, too, were a maze of cuts, and
> each cut represented a chance for blood poisoning.
> Some worked at the stamping machines, and it was
> very seldom that one could work long there at the
> pace that was set, and not give out and forget himself
> and have a part of his hand chopped off . . . and as
> for the other men, who worked in tank rooms full of
> steam, and in some of which there were open vats
> near the level of the floor, their peculiar trouble was
> that they fell into the vats; and when they were fished
> out, there was never enough of them left to be worth
> exhibiting,—sometimes they would be overlooked for
> days, till all but the bones of them had gone out to the
> world as Durham's Pure Leaf Lard![53]

The fear of human lard in American pantries led to legislation on
meatpacking and food inspections. Sinclair was disappointed, though.
He had hoped for workplace reforms, an end to exploitative "wage
slavery," and a political groundswell that would right the evils of brute
capitalism and herald a humane, socialist future. Instead, he got the
Food and Drug Administration. As he said himself, "I aimed at the
public's heart, and by accident I hit it in the stomach."

◆ Cuchulainn Defeated? ◆

The nineteenth century wasn't only iron and steam. It was Gamgee and
Bakewell, inoculations and selective breeding. It was industrial manu-
facturing applied to meat and milk, intensive land use, the feeding of

the maximum number of animals for the maximum gain in carcass yield. When the longhorns died, so did the use of cattle as jack-of-all-beasts. The new Texas beeves were no longer treated like animals, but as canned goods.

Ecology doesn't understand annual growth charts and international market demands. Nor does business understand that floods, plagues, and droughts are an ecosystem's ways of keeping species in balance with their world. What business does understand is that a fourteen-hundred-pound steer is worth more than a seven-hundred-pound one, especially if it's been fed cheaply, takes up little ground, and lives for a mere sixteen months before slaughter. And that's where business started to go wrong.

Cowboys left a cultural legacy far disproportionate to their numbers, their achievements, or their economic impact. To list all the cowboy movies, musical acts, clothing lines, and political apery would take a compendium of monstrous, even Texan, proportions, and to analyze its meaning would require a rawhide Baudrillard. Suffice to say that in large parts of America, a Stetson is equivalent to a monk's tonsure—it's a badge of belief. Instead of believing in the holy apostolic church, though, its wearers believe in "individualism," in steel guitars, and in nostalgia for the open prairie.

A curious coda on the long drive is the renaissance of professional bull riding. Rodeo sports—the reenactments of cattlemen's skills like roping steers and riding broncos—have been a fringe sport in the United States for a century. To the casual eye, rodeo (or "cowboy sports") is less a game than a couture statement. It's a celebration of a Western (and South American) ideal of manhood: tight-buttocked, as grim as a Spartan, and cool enough to not only enter a ring with a giant, bucking animal, but to want to sit on it.

Out of the major cowboy sports, bull riding is the biggest and most life-threatening, the one panting from the heat of its own testosterone. The premise is brutally simple: tie a strap around a bull's sensitive region, then sit on it while it hurls itself around the arena like a two-thousand-pound squash ball, all the while holding one hand up in a gesture of insouciance. If you can last for eight seconds, you win a score, like an ice dancer. It's terribly hard on the bones. Hence the Professional Bull Riders, Inc. motto (which sounds a mere syllable away from being a detergent slogan): "The Toughest Sport on Dirt."

If Spanish bullfighting is about courting death, then American rodeo is about taming life. And marketing. The Professional Bull Riders (PBR) official press kit trumpets its: "pulsating music, expert announcers . . . and production surprises . . . like lasers, . . . pyrotechnics, the Blue Man Group, and featured recording artists such as Jewel." It costs $250,000 to stage such a bull-riding event. Annual prize money—handed out under the arena lights in cowpoke towns like Uncasville, Connecticut, and Las Vegas—is above $11 million. Annual growth in television viewership is a raucous 19.17 percent, reaching more than 104 million consumers with messages from sponsors like Ford Trucks, Wrangler, Jack Daniels, Bud Light, and the U.S. Army.

The bulls themselves are Herculean inventions, being bred, like the toros bravos, especially for sport. Unlike Pedro Trapote's animals, which are weaned to attack, bucking bulls come from stock-breeding programs designed to coax out an instinct for furious thrashing. Naturally, it's a big business. PBR bulls cost up to $100,000 and, since they're not skewered at the climax of the show, and since this is America, they can ascend to celebrity. Mossy Oak Mudslinger, a feted champion, appears on toys and children's apparel and lends his likeness to a coin-operated "kiddie ride" at Wal-Mart.

It's a long way from the long drive. But then, the rise and fall of the cattle drive was always about money, not sentiment. Nostalgia's place is in the poetry book:

> An ancient long-horned bovine
> Lay dying by the river;
> There was a lack of vegetation
> And the cold winds made him shiver;
> A cowboy sat beside him,

With sadness in his face,
To see his final passing,—
This last of a noble race.
    The ancient eunuch struggled
And raised his shaking head,
Saying, "I care not to linger
When all my friends are dead.
These Jerseys and these Holsteins,
They are no friends of mine;
They belong to the nobility
Who live across the brine.
    "Tell the Durhams and the Herefords
When they come a-grazing round,
And see me lying stark and stiff
Upon the frozen ground,
I don't want them to bellow
When they see that I am dead,
For I was born in Texas,
Near the river that is Red.
    "Tell the coyotes, when they come at night,
A-hunting for their prey,
They might as well go further,
For they'll find it will not pay:
If they attempt to eat me
They very soon will see
That my bones and hide are petrified,—
They'll find no beef on me.
    "I remember in the seventies,
Full many summers past,
There was grass and water plenty,
But it was too good to last.
I little dreamed what would happen
Some twenty summers hence,

When the nester came with his wife, his kids,
His dogs, and the barbed-wire fence."

—From "The Last Longhorn"
attributed to John Wesley,
ca. 1899[54]

◆ Carnivore ◆

The tinny smell of old blood hangs on Narok like a veil, trapping in the flies. It comes from scores of shops hung with warm, raw beef, suspended from hooks by the windows. The smell is sour with yellow grease, but it isn't exactly rotten. To a Western nose, sheltered by cellophane and refrigerants, the smell is as strong as a cigar in a closet. A visitor comes to recognize the smell as synonymous with the Masai.

On the morning that Jerry took us to the slaughterhouse, the smell was already thickening in the pools of sunlight outside the storefronts. He drove hard up a broken road out of the town, passing single cows, and dogs gnawing their secrets in the grass. The slaughterhouse road was one of Jerry's regular commutes. In addition to his professions as a veterinarian, a vectorborne disease control officer, an ex-chess prodigy, and a luminary at the nonprofit Maasai Education Discovery organization, Jerry was a government meat inspector.

He sharked our jeep through a bumpy pasture toward a colorless square building about the size of an auto shop. A gang of cheerful-looking cow dealers in street clothes stood at the open loading doors watching six butchers finish skinning a headless animal. Severed horns littered the grass. Whereas the old blood smell in Narok had been powerful, here the reek of viscera was stunning.

Jerry shook a half-dozen hands, then roared, "Hey, you! Get out of there! You can't walk in there dressed like that!"

Parting the crowd like grass, he charged to the door and hauled out a pair of shamefaced Masai wearing baseball caps and jeans. "Put on a white coat and boots!" bellowed Jerry. "It's not hygienic!"

The slaughterhouse operator wasn't a Masai, but a Luhya named Charles Sikoya, from the Lake Victoria region. He was grave, over-worked, and possessed a perfectly spherical head. Since the slaughter-house had no electricity, and thus no refrigeration, the business of dressing the carcasses and loading them into the butchers' trucks had to be done quickly. It was Sikoya's job to see it through without any gross breaches of food-handling regulation. This was hard to do. A knot of patient women sat on rocks outside the slaughterhouse's side door, watching the butchers as intently as a dog will watch a forkful of food poised above its master's plate. The butchers were dumping blood and viscera, but occasionally a woman would approach, a plastic shop-ping bag held tight.

"Gumboot meat," grunted Jerry. "The butchers drop meat into their boots and sell it out the door. It's stealing." He shook his head. "I will have to come back here next week and spend some time getting things in order."

There was no pretense in the work here, no facades that there was anything afoot except the extermination and dismemberment of ani-mals. Cows walked singly up a ramp that led into an unlit chamber. A hatch closed behind them, one at a time, and a worker shot a bolt into the back of their skulls. Still upright, a wall opened, and the stunned animal dropped on its side, whereupon another worker cut its throat, bleeding it into a funnel. From there, a team of workers sliced open the midsection, hauled out the intestines and stomach, and then raised the carcass on ropes for skinning and decapitation. They handled about fifteen cows every morning.

There was a commotion at the front of the building as a worker in gory robes climbed onto the back of a pickup truck and started swing-ing red joints into a metal locker. The woman butcher whom we had seen at the cattle market stood, arrestingly primped, at the side of the truck, an unreal swathe of pleated beige and gray among the blood-stains. The gumboot ladies looked, by contrast, as wild and lively as parakeets.

"It's always a gamble, because some animals have a lot of blood," said Jerry. "She bought her cattle yesterday, judging their live weight by looking at them. But you never know how much meat will come out."

We took a cup of wincingly sugary chai in the corrugated iron snack bar next to the slaughterhouse. Cattle traders with long, distended earlobes ate sweet buns off tin plates and complained about interest rates. On a good day, a trader can make 2,000 shillings on the sale of a cow—approximately $30. They may sell five cows per week. One of Jerry's disciples, a trader and cattle farmer named Olemasyar, told us that his last sale to the Kenyan meat commission netted him a 35 percent loss. Not surprisingly, Olemasyar was a gloomy fellow.

We drove into town with him and lunched in the courtyard of a boardinghouse on Narok's main road. The smell of old blood was especially pungent here—a raw side of meat hung on a hook just inside the entranceway, yellowing in the afternoon heat. A waiter brought us a tray of boiled beef ends that looked gray and stringy, but the flavor, far from being rancid, was merely condensed, with a smack of iron. Jerry explained that the owner of the boardinghouse had sold off his cattle, bought property, and then bought his cattle back with the rent money.

"That is what people need to do," said Jerry. "Sell off their stock and build houses. Cattle can die. A house, you can keep forever."

Olemasyar, whose earlobes drooped proudly to his shoulders, had three wives and a hundred cattle. He talked, unemotionally, about droughts, losses, and the inevitable decay of Masai tradition. He wanted his kids to be politicians and lawyers, even if it meant them moving away. Even if it meant them no longer living like Masai.

"In the traditional way of thinking," he said, "you do what you must today to survive. It's centered on livestock. There's no planning for the future." He shrugged. "That can't go on, and people have to accept it."

On our last night in Nairobi, we drove through the enveloping murk of the deep, inky gaps between streetlights. African electricity doesn't flow in a grid, but bubbles up, like marsh gas, around islands of money. The rest is dark and hooded with trees. So while the Carnivore restaurant blooms with wattage—incandescent reds and violets and golden yellows in every nook, like an irradiated flower bed—the parking lot requires the use of flashlights.

We had come here for our farewell dinner, as had every other foreigner in Kenya with a plane ticket for the next morning. The Carnivore is as ingrained on the tourist itinerary as the airport bureau d'exchange or a photo with a Colobus monkey. A dozen buses shuddered and gusted while their inmates huddled for souvenir pictures by the tamarind plants. They all looked plump under their T-shirts, sweating goodwill and alcohol.

Jerry led us through a maw of carved pillars and toward a round stone grill bristling with iron skewers hung with the impaled parts of sheep. Ranks of sausages browned and dribbled. Haunches and sirloins twisted in the heat. Chicken skins fizzed with grease. The servers wore zebra-striped aprons and carried whole turkeys spitted on swords. Everywhere we saw a theme-park jumble of stuffed lions, heartwood timber, and modern restrooms polished like diamonds, with never a chirp of Swahili to be heard unless the waiters serenaded a birthday party with a chorus from *The Lion King*. It's deservedly the most famous restaurant in Africa.

Jerry, though as companionable as ever ("The problem with Nairobi is that people don't help each other. Just the other day, a thug tried to grab the watch off my wrist. I had to beat him up, as well as four of his friends . . ."), seemed reserved, even sapped. It had been a rough, dusty drive from Narok that morning, and the Nairobi traffic had surpassed its customary viciousness. Apart from the restaurant staff, Jerry's was one of the few black faces in the dining room.

When we had parked our jeep in the darkness outside, he had pointed over a tangle of shrubs, toward the highway.

"That's Kibera over there," he had said. "The biggest slum in East Africa. They have a lot of problems. No water. No electricity. Disease is a big problem. So are gangs. It's very bad." We had been reading daily accounts of violence in Kibera—decapitations were the flavor of the season. But Jerry dropped the subject and we went inside to eat.

We chewed for an hour, commenting solely on the food. Chicken livers, ostrich balls, Chinese spareribs, and roasts of every barnyard denizen except for the cat. A waiter carved a beef rump at swordpoint, about half an inch thick. Then came lamb. And sausage. And turkey. And more beef. No storied gluttons—not Lucullus, not Henry VIII, not even Elvis—had ever swamped themselves with so many pounds of flesh. We ate our way past satiety and into hazy tracts into stupor.

6

THE $300 SIRLOIN

*Cattle in the Twentieth and
Twenty-first Centuries*

◆ Death *of a* Small-Town Butcher ◆

There's a pathos to dead Victorian cities, less wistful than the melancholy in older, fallen places. It has to do with the architecture—the squat brick estates surrounding grandiose libraries, bathhouses, and banks shaped by industrialists' love of aped Gothic. It also has to do with the spirit of the workhouse, of the toil and hunger behind the sepia photographs of people with proud eyes and big moustaches. And it has to do with the soot. In the West Yorkshire city of Bradford, once the wool capital of the world, the grime seeped into the gritstone a hundred years ago and never left. But most of the people have.

Bradford's city hall is a florid monument, if not to hubris, than to presumption. Designed in the 1860s and erected out of an unshakable belief in flying buttresses and wool money, it's a monster's confection;

a stone fancy spindled with life-size statues of every English monarch from William the Conqueror to Victoria. The builders even invoked the Florentine Medicis with a massive, tumescent clock tower modeled on the one in the Palazzo Vecchio, topped with scrolling ironwork, an unwise amount of gold trim, and thirteen bells installed for the princely sum of £5,000. Bradford's city fathers, in 1869, were confident men.

A hundred years later the bells stood silenced, unrung for fear of shattering their rotten wooden frames. Public restoration grants have since given them safe housings, but there aren't many ears left to hear the chimes. The wool barons are long gone. Tourists don't stop much. Economic despair doesn't sell in the guidebooks, and you can't decently call a boarded shopfront or litter-strewn thoroughfare "quaint" or a "hidden treasure." On a Sunday afternoon, even the Anglican cathedral is locked and abandoned, and although its lawns are neatly mown, from its grounds you can see a crest of derelict housing towers. One is par-ticularly grim: a Soviet-type oblong, bisected by wrecking balls, leaving a gap in the skyline like a missing tooth. Hallways yawn into air and bedrooms are laid open like the rooms in a dollhouse, save for the wild spaghetti of ripped electrical cables spewing out of the split cement. But there are no cranes or demolition crews on hand to complete the job. Bradford doesn't even have the energy to finish burying itself.

One of Bradford's lost souls is Colin Beaumont, formerly a butcher who sidelined in carryout roasts and meat pies. Outside of the British Commonwealth, the meat pie is a quiet source of puzzlement—it's hard to imagine a gang of Americans watching football and cracking beers over hot steak and kidney. This neglect is unjust. Yorkshire's pies are delightful. Beef pies are made of salty gobbets suspended in brown gravy that's viscous without being gluey, and the best ones, called "gala pies," traditionally feature not only a mixture of veal and pork but also a whole boiled egg in the center: sort of a cholesterol surprise. York-shire butchers take their pies very seriously. They compete for honors in annual bake-offs, during which virgin pie eaters can be spotted by the brown slicks down the fronts of their shirts. Meat pies, because of their leaden innards, are structurally unsafe.

Although it's as English as a hand-knit tea cozy, these pies embody the Gallic virtues of liberté (it's portable and unconstrained by mealtimes), fraternité (it's the staple lunch of every unionized laborer in Yorkshire), and egalité (a fresh pie costs 80p, or about $1.60). In addition to gala and pure pork pies, the primary varieties are steak and kidney, mince and onions, and beef and potato. Within these basic groupings lies enormous room for nuance. This comes in gravies. Some are sweet, like the "jelly" in the gala pie. Others are sticky and savory, like Bovril syrup. It's in the crust, however, that butchers truly flaunt their skills, kneading the pastry with a girlish tenderness. Delicacy is all, and a heavy hand squeezes out too much air.

Meat pies are often dressed with relishes like sweet Branson Pickle or hot piccalilli—a mustard concoction made of cabbage, cauliflower, onion, and enough vinegar to put a frown on a Buddha. Dried marrowfat peas, boiled into a swampy cream, are another accompaniment (a plastic tub of these "mushy pease" is the only vegetable stalwart enough to brave the shelves of most West Yorkshire butchers' shops). The meal should be taken with milky "builder's tea" steeped strong in the mug. If West Yorkshire has a flavor, it's the melded aromas of beef pie, mushy peas, and teabags.

B eaumont described his butcher's life over a dinner of beef Wellington, the filling of which came from cows on a farm lying less than a hundred miles distant.[1] He recounted dark mornings rolling dough with his wife, Alison, and long days working the cleaver and till.

"Every day, old ladies are coming in, year after year, buying for their husbands. Nineteen sixties men, right?" said Beaumont. The Wellington was as tender as jelly, and we drank Tetley's West Yorkshire bitter while he reminisced about the old ladies' clockwork visits: Monday, steak and kidneys; Tuesdays, liver and onions. "You could see them looking in the window and before they'd even come into the shop, have their things ready for them, right regular every day. During haying season, farm wives would be in buying for the men in the fields, things like an entire shoulder for sandwiches."

The Beaumonts felt as established as the village church, and considerably more popular. They were a human link between people and the animals they ate, a shortening loop in a chain that's grown longer as we've distanced ourselves from our food.

Then, in Scotland in the 1990s, steak pie laced with *E. coli* killed five people. The butchers, said the press, were to blame. A flurry of new health codes legislated expensive monitoring equipment, more inspections, and the costly uprooting of traditional white tiles that once lined the cutting rooms (grout is a nest for bacteria). And that was before mad cow disease terrified the public with the specter of a murderous hamburger.

The coup de grâce came when a rash of foot-and-mouth disease shut down the English countryside for months, robbing the butchers of any meats more romantic than chicken and sausages. As always, it was the small shops, the county slaughterhouses, and the village farms that perished. Supermarket chains weathered the blow by buying meat from across the country, or from Europe, while the disease ruined local operations. "Must have been close on a hundred butchers in Bradford," said Beaumont. "Now, can't think of one in the town center."

All the dangers campaigned against by Gamgee in the nineteenth century—and that his successors, forgetting the lessons of rinderpest, ignored during the twentieth—had converged on West Yorkshire. Beaumont sold out, as have tens of thousands of other butchers in the generation since people discovered cholesterol.[2]

Colin, unlike his native Bradford, adapted to the economic jolts of his times. He laid down his cleaver and raised a hammer, training himself for the much more lucrative work of renovating scenic Yorkshire barns into country homes for rich Londoners. He was the adaptive iguana, changing his skin according to the demands of circumstance. His city, however, proved to be a dodo. When the wool trade went extinct, so did Bradford's prosperity. The city never embraced Darwin's lesson of reinvention or death.

◆ Two Dodos ◆
The Beef *and* Milk Industries Today

Like Bradford in the nineteenth century, the American beef and dairy businesses are clumsy, overweight, and waddling toward a very nasty encounter with the modern world. Their problem is design. In both, profits come from dumping oceans of milk and Alpine mounds of meat into the shopping carts of a thoughtless public. Reduce the volume, and the profits vanish into millions of tons of carefully engineered (and genetically modified) feed. The industry's economics mean it has to be big, and it has to be stable. If anything rattles its volume-profit axis, say if a drought hits the cornfields that feed the animals, then the whole thing is upended in the dust. The year 2008 was especially dire. Grain prices zoomed upward partly due to international demands for bio-ethanol and for animal feed in the Chinese and Indian markets, and on account of a miserly wheat harvest in Australia. But mostly due to the leap in the cost of oil, which resonates in every line of a grain farmer's budget, from fertilizer to irrigation to harvesting and transport, cattle farmers reliant on grain are feeling queasy. Likewise, while the industry assumes that consumers will always buy inexpensive cow products, they would prefer that we neither taste nor think about what we're swallowing. Too much introspection is a bad thing, and many Americans, through financial necessity or apathy, are willing to oblige. But the industry, like wool-boom Bradford, is built on the presumption that the universe is static.

There are, of course, critics. Among the cubes and squiggles of London's Tate Modern Gallery, there's a picture of what appear to be two meat cleavers lying, side by side, on mustard. A twentieth-century painter called Peter Kinley was responsible, and his two cleavers, which are no more than two brown rectangles with little handles, are called *Two Cows*. The rectangles are, of course, the featureless bodies of the animals, and the handles are their unnecessary heads. They're as identical as microchips, while their background trades Gainsborough's

green and living tangles for a uniform yellow wash. Kinley has reduced
the British landscape to lumps of geometry, just as in the last half century we've reduced cattle to their constituent steaks. On *Two Cows*,
Kinley said, "I have . . . painted animals . . . to reassert, among other
things, their right to respect in a culture which I believe accords them
only marginal consideration."[3]

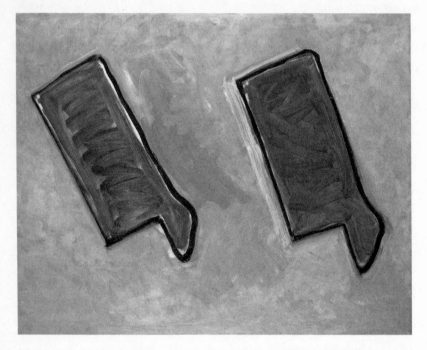

TWO COWS BY PETER KINLEY, 1981. *Credit: © Catherine
Kinley. Courtesy Osborne Samuel Ltd, London.*

"Marginal consideration" is a generous phrase. A huge industry is
devoted to deconstructing these animals into less than the sums of
their bodies. There's a cost to seeing life in squares.

In 2002, about ninety-eight million cows lived in the United States,
of which 10 percent belonged to the dairy herd.[4] The rest were beef
cows that spent their youth on one of the country's eight hundred
thousand small, and generally family-run, "cow-calf" farms. There
they lived traditional lives. They wandered the pastures, suckling at

their mothers' teats before being weaned to grass. And they ate a lot of this. So much, indeed, that within about a year they inflated to the weight of 650 pounds, at which point they made the jump to the industrial feedlot.

These are big operations. In some cases, shockingly big. USDA figures say that in 2002 there were about twenty-two hundred feedlots with herds numbering above a thousand head, and a handful that boasted as many as one hundred thousand animals. To conscientious consumers, the reputation of these operations is now something of a cross between the Third Circle of Hell and a discount drugstore. The animals huddle in concrete pens and feed on high-calorie feed that is designed to max out their ability to metabolize protein. Within months, they wax by some four-hundred-odd pounds of marbled muscle. Then they're moved to a packing plant and killed.

This two-stage process (stage one, taking the cow from birth through a youth spent grazing outdoors on a grass diet; stage two, "finishing" it on grain at a feedlot) is an invention of the past half century. Until the 1950s, feedlots scarcely existed, and most American cows spent their entire lives "on grass," as they have evolved to do. Then, around the same time that scientists began flinging metal balls into orbit and packing nuclear fusion reactions into bombs, laboratories hatched up new, high-yielding breeds of corn. Better corn, coupled with the flowering toxicity of new pesticides, a blooming fruitfulness in chemical fertilizers, and a steely fleet of deep-bladed tractors, meant that corn shot up like wildfire across the Midwest. It was the Great Corn Boom, and the intensive cattle industry exists because of it. Until recently, America floundered in an ocean of cheap grain that weighed down the commodities markets with the same lumpish plenitude that weighs down our midriffs. For decades we've grown too much corn. We couldn't eat all of it. Africa couldn't afford it. Europe didn't need it. Asia prefers rice. So agriculturalists began unloading the surplus calories on cows.

Enter the hundred-thousand-head feedlot. Along with better vaccines and breeding programs that invoked the ghost of Robert Bakewell,

farmers could now breed legions of gargantuan cows. The economy of
scale ballooned. In the past fifteen years alone, the number of American cattle farms dropped by 16 percent, even as the number of cattle
remained stable.[5] These changes have almost all occurred in the feedlot
or finishing industry. The cow-calf ranch that takes the animal from
birth through to the end of its first year of life (plus or minus a month
depending on the market, rainfall, and the breed) is still a regular feature in the American countryside. The feedlots, however, have exploded
in size, have become geographically concentrated (Kansas and Arizona
host a third of the country's feedlots, raising three-quarters of its beef),
and are the source of many of today's worries about the ethics, welfare,
and sustainability of meat.

The dangers of this system are legion.[6] To boost corn yield, soil is
leached of water, nitrogen, potassium, and phosphorus. Feedlots spew
lakes of manure. The internal organs of the animals themselves, which
evolved to eat grass, are ruined by being crammed with grain. Controversial antibiotics and hormones keep these huge concentrations of
animals clean of bugs, at least, but there's no pleasant way to think
about their final journeys in crammed cattle trucks. Of course, these
ecological and animal welfare offenses, to say nothing of potential
health effects on consumers, pall in the light of our national right to a
cheap lunch.

⌘

CULINARY INTERLUDE

The American Hamburger

Knead 1½ pounds ground round or chuck with 3 tablespoons white
bread crumbs, one-fourth of a grated onion, 2 tablespoons tomato
juice, 3 teaspoons Worcestershire sauce, 1 teaspoon garlic powder, and
salt and pepper. Mold meat into four or five symmetrical wads. Grill or
fry in an oiled skillet about five minutes per side, or seven if a drier
burger is desired. Consistency should be yielding, but not pasty, and

the juices from the meat should flow. Serve on a toasted bun, and accent with sliced vegetables, guacamole, or melted cheese.

Cheap meat is no small addiction. Cattle have pricked at humanity's appetites throughout our evolutionary and historical journeys, so to dismiss our greed for beef as an irrational vice, fixed by a stern poster on the classroom wall, would be as useful as denying the libido. That's why we've invented industrial cattle production—to satisfy desire. Like most businesses that traffic in passions, it mirrors a darker aspect of the human character, one that, as long as it's gorged, doesn't worry about consequences. The milking trade is hardly different.

To see just how distorted the dairy industry is today, it's helpful to look at the past. American painter John Steuart Curry (1897–1946) captured something of a snapshot of the old pasturelands in *Wisconsin Landscape*, his image of a utopia of grass fields, barns, woodlots, and hay bales, offsetting a comfortable black-and-white streak of Holstein-Frisians. The barn is brightly painted. Water flows clear. It's likely that the unseen farmer has a strong jaw, a bible, and a brood of flaxen-haired tots, squeaky clean except for fingers sticky with Mom's apple pie. Only above, in a sky muddy with rain clouds, is there dissonance.

Viewed from more prosaic eyes, we see a picture of a working farm in which locally grown hay is drying for winter feed, while roaming dairy animals have their way with the landscape. So far, so bucolic. But then, the painting was made in the late 1930s, at the gasping end of the Depression. Farmers in Wisconsin were, on the whole, a wretched bunch. But Curry was peddling dreams, soft comforts. His purpose is therapeutic, and paintings like this one provide the means for "spiritual and cultural rejuvenation, pointing back toward traditional values that could lead the nation out of its crisis."[7]

Curry could never have rejuvenated spirits by painting a picture of a modern milking barn. Although Wisconsin is still a haven for small-scale dairies—today's average herd is only 59 cows per farm, well below the U.S. national average of 120 cows per farm[8]—the trend is toward the gigantic, particularly in California.[9] On the West Coast, herds of 1,000, to 2,000 animals are not uncommon,[10] and, in 1999, averaged 530 Holstein-Frisians—the breed that makes up 90 percent of American and European dairy cows.[11] Consolidation has meant that California dairies went from producing 8 percent of American milk in 1970 to 18 percent in 1998. In short, the typical quart of American milk comes from an increasingly large herd. If you live on the West Coast, then your milk probably comes from a herd in which most of its members have probably never seen one another.

Each animal is milked at least two times a day to produce up to thirty liters of milk. This isn't very healthy. Rates of mastitis—an infection of the teat—and lameness, which are entirely preventable if farmers are attuned to the needs of their animals, are rising. Four in ten cows get mastitis each year. Life expectancy, which used to be about twenty-five years, is falling. Regardless of their health, most dairy cows are slaughtered after about five years, the point at which their productivity begins to wane. Furthermore, like the feedlot industry for beef, these large dairy systems are an environmental disaster. To feed these legions of milk-producing animals, grain specially grown for the purpose needs to be transported in colossal bulk—burning proportionate fossil fuels. Mountains of manure poison and clog the groundwater.

Between the two of them, feedlots and huge dairy herds are brutalizing the environment. The Food and Agriculture Organization of the United Nations goes so far as to accuse the global livestock industry of spewing more greenhouse gases than does the world's transportation fleet. It also says that cattle—again due to feedlots and large milking parlors—are sucking up our water. Adult beef cows produced in feedlots drink eleven liters of water per day. Dairy cows that are kept indoors and fed only grain drink twenty-two liters. By contrast, pastured animals need about five liters of water, since they're hydrated by eating moist grass.[12]

The crippling costs in water, fuel, and feed should be enough to worry the industry, and they are. Feed costs are rising by staggering degrees. Ledgers are awash in red. According to Jeff Stolle, vice president of marketing for the Nebraska Cattlemen, Nebraska cattle feeders are spending an extra $5 million a day on feed.[13] But it usually takes an act of God to cause a panic. In nineteenth-century Bradford, no one thought to spread the economic risk by balancing the city's skewed reliance on the wool trade. Only when the bottom dropped from the market in the late nineteenth century did people notice how fragile their fortunes had really been. Acts of God, of course, are almost always predictable.

Here's a brief list of potential calamities: a disease in the production chain, a drought that cuts grain supply, rising fuel costs, pathogens, antipollution taxes, foreign competition, unexpected hazards from cloning, and even the possibility that consumers suddenly take fright, perhaps accepting the antimeat rhetoric that their favorite food may be steeped in hormones and antibiotics.

Any of these could spoil the industry's revenues, and, given a few bad years, could push it into the deep, red ink ocean of unprofitability. That's what happened to the wool trade. And that's what bled Bradford in a hundred-year death. The cattle industry is likely to go quicker. It doesn't take a century to die of thirst.

◆ A Dry Future ◆

The literature of desiccation has a fertile history. The Book of Genesis says that the earth lay barren until God summoned up a divine mist from the ground, muddying the dirt into a gloop from which he molded Adam. Celtic myth is riddled with stories of questing heroes in dry wastelands. They became Christianized in the Arthurian cycle with the story of Sir Percival and the ailing Fisher King, and made a final transition to metaphor when T. S. Eliot described the collapse as: "This is the dead land / This is cactus land."

On the human plane, Coleridge's Ancient Mariner first croaked the line, "Water, water everywhere, nor any drop to drink," but fresh water is the motive in a vast corpus of maritime and shipwreck literature spanning Homer to Patrick O'Brian. An overlooked trifle from the great Irish humorist Flann O'Brien is *Thirst*, a one-act sketch about a bartender describing a hot day on the King's Service in Mesopotamia: "There we were, staggerin' through the bloody . . . boilin'— blanketty-blank heat. . . . And the worst of it—a hot, dry thirst comin' up . . . like the blast from a furnace." O'Brien's play ends with a clarion call to rally around the beer tap. On a geographical, and indeed spiritual level, however, John Steinbeck is the bard of thirsty ground: "Often I was so full of dust that I drove blind . . . But I kept driving on and on, by guess and instinct. I was making my last stand in the Dust Bowl."[14]

A repeat of a 1930s Dust Bowl is imminent. A drought will happen. The cattle industry isn't ready for it.

The year 2005–2006 was fairly dry. First, dry weather in the United States and Australia (and Iraq's reemergence on the world scene as an importer of wheat) started to drive wheat prices up. Feedlot farmers stopped buying wheat and upped the proportions of corn and soybeans they fed to their animals. This, of course, triggered a rise in corn prices, and, with feed costs escalating, cattle farmers saw the "breakeven" price, the price they have to sell at to recover costs, rising by $5 to $6. Since this break-even price for yearling cattle is around $80 or $90, a $5 jolt is grave.[15]

Light rainfall in 2005 meant less water to drink. Unable to keep their calves on pasture, ranchers sold stock ahead of schedule, lost money on the deal, and swelled the crowded feedlots with ever more beef. The feedlot operators couldn't afford to buy enough corn for their stock, so they slaughtered them young, upping beef production in the first quarter of 2006 by 6.4 percent above the previous year. Americans ate it up and, buoyed by cut-rate T-bones, farmers survived another year. But their operating margins thinned.

It's the pattern, not an individual bad season, that's the problem. Dry weather means ranchers sell their stock early, feedlot operators sell their animals before they reach full maturity, and slaughterhouses process a glut of young carcasses. The supermarkets are flush with cheap beef for a few months, but the stability of the whole industry takes another jostle.

Compared with the days of Steinbeck's choking clouds on the prairies, 2005–2006 passed in moistened comfort. Since the Dust Bowl at least two severe droughts parched the land east of the Rockies—much of which is classified as "semiarid." The rains failed in 1951–1956, halving the crop yield in large areas of Kansas, Texas, and other grainlands. Again, dry weather in 1987–1989 cost the American economy an estimated $39 billion.[16] At the time, it was the country's most expensive natural disaster to date.

The Dust Bowl even happened before the Dust Bowl. Paleoclimatology, the study of historic climate changes, uses the thickness of tree rings and the types of salt in the sediment at the bottom of lakes to reconstruct ancient rainfall data. For example, by plumbing the sludge at the bottom of Moon Lake in North Dakota, scientists have learned that the past three hundred years were relatively sodden. From A.D. 200–400, and again between 600–700 and 1000–1200, the region felt consecutive, protracted droughts.[17] Douglas fir trees in New Mexico, which can live for more than a thousand years, prove that the twentieth century is a damp patch in a dusty timeline. North America eight hundred years ago would have been a mess of brushfires, skinny bison, and roving, careworn people. But the native prairie was able to withstand natural cycles of drought. A knotty mass of roots lay under the soil, trapping water. Countless species of perennial grasses meant that if one type withered, there were replacements, and since grass is a tough plant, it could usually revive even after a long stretch between drinks. Grain fields are comparative wimps. They need annual plowing and seeding, and they let most of their water supply dribble past their feeble roots.

Since the modern American landscape is meshed with fences, sunbaked animals aren't free to walk to wetter pastures. Locked into their acreage, ranchers can't let their cattle roam like the bison of yore, snuffling out forage and water holes during a dry spell. They're forced to sell their animals or let them die. Grain farmers, too, are at the mercy of the thermometer. As climate change gathers steam, the northerly prairies, especially in Canada, are beginning to enjoy a longer grain-growing period, and a shorter blast of frost in the winter. But the southern part of the grain belt can't sustain the longer growing period. Plants will lose more moisture through "evapotranspiration"—having the water baked out of them in the heat—and the soil won't be able to replace the extra fluid.

It's not all bad news. Citrus farmers may see a golden, frost-free future. But some climate models suggest a loss of 20 percent of the available surface water on the Great Plains.

Heat, desiccation, and the loss of a fecund fifth of our prime agri-cultural earth. This litany of disaster is boomingly pronounced in the 2001 *Third Assessment Report* of the Intergovernmental Panel on Cli-mate Change (IPCC)—a tome as dire as the blackest utterances of Nostradamus, but scarier on account of the pie charts. Nor is the 2001 report as bad as the *Fourth Assessment Report* published in 2007. In purest oxygen-starved prose, we're warned of "very likely" drought in-creases and possible average temperature boosts of five degrees by 2090. What they're saying is that hell will be unleashed on Topeka.

While this is alarming, the fact remains that we are not polar bears, tied to a diet of seal cubs. In times of hunger, we have always, eventu-ally, scrounged a meal, or found new sources of food. We are adaptable. And therein lies the problem. Cattle farmers are wonderfully attuned to changes in input prices, international commodity markets, and mortgage rates—and they take a lot of trouble to protect themselves against the slings and arrows from these quarters. But they haven't done much about drought.

The reason they're not panicking is irrigation. The Great Plains sit on top of the Ogallala Aquifer, one of the greatest underground bodies of water in the world. As the glaciers melted back toward the Rockies between ten thousand and twenty-five thousand years ago, they trickled and dripped enough fresh water to fill a reservoir underlying 174,000 square miles of farmland. It held three billion-acre feet of water (an acre-foot is the amount of water needed to flood an acre to the depth of one foot, which is about 325,000 gallons). For the past fifty years, this invaluable resource below Wyoming, South Dakota, Nebraska, Kansas, Colorado, Oklahoma, New Mexico, and Texas has been the farmers' safeguard against a rainless summer, or three.

The water lay too deep for Dust Bowl farmers to tap it, which is why their lives blew away in the hot winds. Only in the 1950s, when the automobile industry developed powerful new engines, could pumps finally reach the aquifer. But even when they sucked up the water, they couldn't distribute it over such a vast area. At least not until 1952, when an inventor named Frank Zybach patented the "Zybach Self-Propelled Sprinkling Apparatus." The son of a blacksmith, and a farmer by vocation, Zybach knew the backbreaking labor involved in lugging heavy sprinkler pipes between grain fields. So he attached an arm to a wellhead that held a series of sprinklers, and, after propping the apparatus up on soft rubber tires, used some of the sprinklers' water flow to power the wheels. The result was the world's first self-propelled irrigation system, a miraculous device that allowed farmers to effortlessly soak vast acreages with mist.

Zybach's system turned the Dust Bowl into a breadbasket. Today's sprinklers spray in circles of a half-mile diameter, with liquid fertilizer injected into the pipes for an extra smack of minerals. Satellite-linked computers tailor the level of nutrients and flow of water for each section of crop. In short, Zybach created fields that are immune to drought. Regardless of rainfall, the sprinklers can run all year long.

The problem is, 20 percent of irrigation water in the United States now comes from the Ogallala Aquifer.[18] This is a resource that, like oil, can never be replaced—the Texas Water Development Board says that only 7.4 percent of the pumped water is recharged each year. Since we started tapping the aquifer we've drained it by a third.[19]

Beef feedlots are fed by grain grown in Zybach's irrigated crop circles. When the water dries up, so does the grain, and with the grain goes the entire system of concentrated beef and dairy production. Some grain farmers are reading the forecasts and turning off their sprinklers, switching back to less thirsty crops, like wheat instead of corn.[20] But there isn't a choice left for beef farmers. Their utility bills, more so than the dust clouds outside their office windows, will force them to close the feedlots. They're going to have to change. Perhaps not right away—there's always insurance, government emergency aid, and selling off stock, or even farmland. But change they must.

The most significant shift has to be mental. In the beef business, this means exorcising the ghost of Robert Bakewell and forswearing the style of intensive cattle farming that's kept meat on every lunch plate in America for half a century. As producers, they're going to have to adapt a leaner economic model. As consumers, we're going to have to learn something unnatural to the American character: restraint.

Restraint has been the mantra of environmentalists since the dying days of the passenger pigeon, but the most effective tool for forcing Americans to rethink their habits is to raise prices. With lower beef production, this will happen anyway. The real question is how to remodel the industry itself, so that it's profitable, sustainable, and capable of filling the millions of hamburger buns left vacant by the shuttered feedlots. This is hardly easy. Industries as complex as the cattle business take time to shift course. For example, between 1967 and 1979, a raft of troubles—ranging from government policies to drought—squeezed cattle farmers between high costs and low beef prices. But despite economic woes, the cattle population actually grew from 110 million head in 1967 to 130 million in 1975. Animals aren't widgets; you can't change the level of cattle production to match the month's financial numbers. Living creatures take time to be born, grow up, and get pregnant. Only in 1979 did the number of cattle finally drop back to a manageable 110 million.

The industry itself sees stormy waters on the horizon. Even before the current crisis of high feed costs, cattlemen saw that while beef prices were rising, profits were not. "Margins are thin," says Kevin Good, a senior marketing analyst at Cattle Fax, a beef industry information service. "There's excess capacity and land values are escalating. There are a lot of things you can do with land that's more profitable than raising cows on it." Crop production, for example, but also urban development and fishing and shooting reserves. And then there's the price of oil. "Input costs are going up faster than beef prices," says Good, meaning that even today, ranchers are losing money. Good says that the future lies in consolidation, in raising more cows on less land—exactly the opposite of a sustainable plan.

◆ The Criollo Solution ◆

The cardinal virtue of dung is that, when dropped by a cow, it converts back into grass. Once upon a preindustrial epoch, cows were at the center of this virtuous natural cycle that turned grass into dung and dung into more grass, a particularly useful event in places too barren to grow crops. During this epoch, people ate what they could produce without frenetically whisking animals across the face of the planet. Agricultural land chirped, bloomed, and belched with the throngs of nature—the blazing universe of grasses and weeds and partridges that we now lump under the turgid heading "biodiversity." Industrialization got rid of all that.

The story of modernity is the story of that loss. An American philosopher named Wendell Berry once argued that the industrial mindset has taken the solution—by which he meant a life molded by the confines of nature—and divided it neatly into a string of social and environmental problems. There couldn't be a better summary of the cattle industry. Its unwavering pursuit of cheap meat and milk has bred a host of twenty-first-century bugbears: wasteful farming, soil degradation, tsunamis of effluent, and animal welfare offenses. Worse, it's a top-heavy industry with clay feet, reliant on high rainfall and low fuel costs. But the cattle industry, as bloated and ruinous as parts of it are, is itself axiomatic of a much wider perversion.

Cows are animals, and we used to treat them as such. We exploited them alive and dead, but we left them in enough peace so that they could fulfill their life's purpose, which was to stand in a pasture and chew. By yanking them from their habitat, breeding them to physiological extremes, and pushing them through an industrial process as if they were identical to Model Ts, we've forgotten an obvious truth. Being animals, cows are part of an ecological whole, along with the grass and the groundwater. But in the past two hundred years we stopped thinking of cows as living things, and, following the logic of Bakewell to its obvious conclusion, we came to think of them merely as milk wells to be tapped and burgers to be neatly wrapped in polyurethane. We're not arguing that the blessings of modernity haven't been splendid, nourishing billions of people and eradicating the most devilish diseases, to say nothing of luxuries like gas-powered backyard grills, bottled steak sauce, and the rib eye au poivre at Morton's. We're not sounding the Luddite bugle. But it can't last. The cattle industry is not sustainable, at least not in its present form. The first step in making it work better would be to put cows back on grass. A grass diet would mean that feed and water requirements would drop, saving our precious groundwater supplies for that day when the rains stop. On the negative side of the ledger, grass diets are expensive. Or at least they are now. If feed costs continue to rise with the price of oil, this scale may balance itself.

One beef farmer who's returned to the pastoral ideal is Will Harris, a fifth-generation cowman from Tennessee whose great-grandfather, Captain James Edward Harris (CSA), first took a concern in cattle during the Civil War. As a gentleman, he was forced to provision his cavalry troop out of his own pocket, and he did so by buying steers. He lost both his family's farm and his war, but a relative helped him recover his fortunes by giving him a plot of good grassland, which his descendants work to this day under the name of White Oak Pastures.

"My father and grandfather were real animal husbandmen," says Harris, a gray-haired southerner of the mannerly stamp. "They raised cattle in accordance with nature. There were no industrial tools. No confinement feeding of high-carbohydrate diets or unnatural derivates. When the cattle were ready for harvest, they were harvested right there, and then they were consumed by neighbors."

When Harris took over the operation of the farm, he switched production to an industrial model he learned studying animal science at the University of Georgia. But he began to realize that industrial ideas were bluntly opposed to the husbanding methods practiced by his father. "In animal science," says Harris, "you look to science, to research done by industry and land grant universities. Agronomists are focused on fertility programs, how many tons of forage can be produced per acre. They don't follow to see what happens when the beef is fed to the consumer. It's narrow in scope. Whereas animal husbandry is holistic management, more art than science."

"Holistic management," as insipid as the phrase sounds, is Harris's successful answer to the cattle question. It means a grass diet, for a start, which lends the meat a robust flavor and higher doses of nourishments like beta-carotene, omega-3 fatty acids, and vitamin E (all of America's one million cattle and calf operators begin their cattle on grass—it's only later, in the feedlot, that the animals shift to grain). But holistic management also emphasizes the land over the individual cow, the herd over the tenderloin. Knowing that his profits depend on maintaining the earth in working order, a thoughtful holistic farmer might sow his pastures with Bahia grass, which can survive drought, and rye grasses, which can survive too much rain. Either way the clouds swing, the pasture is secure, particularly when reinforced with modern weather forecasts.

Researchers at the Land Institute in Kansas have shown that holistic farming can not only be profitable, but can actually outproduce industrial-style farms. Productivity, measured as food produced per unit of land, tends to drop as farm size increases. Small farms are proven to be better at raising food. And small farms have to sell to local markets, which lowers the waste incurred in trucking food across the country.

These Kansan researchers have also been meddling with grass. They've shown that pastures planted with perennial grasses don't need annual reseeding and plowing—a tremendous savings of money. No plow also means the root system can thicken, building up organic matter in the soil, which traps moisture and nitrogen, reducing the need for fertilizer. It also traps carbon dioxide—the most dastardly of the greenhouse gasses—by "fixing" the carbon in the ground. So in addition to needing less water and fertilizer, organic-rich soil does its bit to save the atmosphere.

Smaller farm size and mixed grasses are good, but resilient cows are better. We've seen that the United States is swamped with Aberdeen Angus beef cattle and Holstein-Frisian dairy cows. These two breeds, being swollen with flesh and milk, respectively, give the best economic return per dollar of investment. They grow up fast. They're the biggest kids in the class. But they're milquetoasts. They take too many sick days and they fall apart at the first crackle of a heat wave. In the arid twenty-first century, our Frisians will curdle like saucepans of boiling cream.

Forward-thinking farmers are already looking to other breeds, ones that yield less product, but that don't demand air conditioners, lakes of imported water, and batteries of antibiotic shots. The Masai cattle, for instance, don't yield as much milk as do Holstein-Frisians, but they do it without an expensive support network of veterinarians and refrigerator apparatus.[21] In Brazil, farmers are abandoning specialty milk or beef cows for "dual-purpose" cattle. The logic holds that it's better to raise a strong cow, yielding both milk and meat, than it is to breed a wheezing, drugged-up *flojo*, brought low by the weight of its own brisket.

The United Nation's Food and Agriculture Organization says that dual-purpose cattle make up 75 percent of South America's dairy herd, providing 90 percent of its milk. These cows are mongrels, descended from productive but temperamental European cows, heat-resistant

Indian zebu cows, and the rangy criollos bred by the conquistadors. One study looked at twenty Venezuelan herds and found sixty-three different genetic groups, with twelve of the farms being home to ten or more strains living together. Mixed herds consistently outperform thoroughbred European ones in South America largely because the mongrels have higher survival and more fecund reproduction rates in extreme climates. They also eat rougher food and succumb to fewer diseases. Compared with an Aberdeen Angus, they're a cheaper, better investment.

Some American farmers have already taken up the criollo banner. Harris's herd at White Oak Pastures includes "cracker cattle," criollos descended from Spanish animals brought to Florida in the 1500s. Now classified as a "heritage breed," they're cousins to the South American cows that can shrug off both withering blasts of sun and the rapaciousness of mosquitoes. Many other American cattlemen have seen the benefits of heritage breeds—pretty Red Devons, for example, on family farms in New England—that thrive in hard weather, strike picturesque poses on the grass, and command high prices in restaurants.

This isn't to say that interbreeding, natural soil, and small farms can do away with the need for farm management. Cows still need vaccines. Pastures need maintenance. Regardless of how hardy the animal or enduring the grass, there will always be emergencies that can only be met by importing feed or quarantining herds. But over the next century, the holistic cattle farmer will have a much better chance of weathering storms, both real and metaphorical.

When trumpeting the need for change, there's a danger in sounding too shrill. Restraint, not dogma, is important in convincing farmers to adapt new methods. If governments force farmers to close feedlots and pasture all their cattle, there's going to be a temptation to bulldoze rain forests. This isn't a particularly good idea, and the UN estimates that between 2000 and 2010, approximately twenty-four million hectares of forest will be converted to livestock pasture.[22] Feedlots would have, in the scheme of environmental health, been a whole lot better.

There really are no magic bullets, no simple solutions to the demand
that billions of consumers have for cattle. Dr. Lauren Gwin of the
American Grassfed Association sees an uncertain future. "If we tried to
produce the same amount of beef as we do now, all on pasture, I'm not
saying it can't be done," she says. "But I don't think mainstream beef
will shift en masse to grass. This came up in the 1970s, in the Southeast. It didn't work out because the price of grain dropped, and farmers
weren't focused on quality. They just shoved a lot of grass into the
cattle and didn't finish them properly." Low-grade meat, even if it's
sustainable, is still a bad investment.

Today's grass-fed cattle farmers are more attuned to the nuances of
consumer taste, but they still face a problem of geography, or rather of
physics. There are only so many fourteen-hundred-pound cows you
can fit on an acre of grass. "The short answer is that it costs more to
raise cattle on grass because the land requirement is great," says Harris.
Or it costs more at the moment. Feedlots are built on an assumption of
cheap grain. Recent government ethanol programs have driven corn
prices up, and look to continue to do so far into the century. But it's
still unnaturally cheap to stuff a cow with corn.

"We've got highly subsidized grain production in this country,"
says Gwin. "But if we kick out the false props, and if it weren't so artificially cheap, they wouldn't raise cattle this way."

Feedlots are, in a very real way, spawn of the U.S. Department of
Agriculture. Without farming subsidies, grain would never have replaced grass as the entrée of choice for America's favorite ruminant. In
Argentina today—a country committed to pampas beef—there's a
shift under way toward feedlots, solely because of government subsidies to grain farmers.[23] It's a worrying thought to anyone who's ever
felt transcendence in a grass-feed steak churrasco with a bottle of
Malbec, but that's the price of funding the corn industry.

Another problem faces grass-fed producers. Gwin observes that
Americans, unlike Argentines and Southern Europeans, prefer the soft
taste of grain-finished beef compared to the vigorous flavor of range
cattle, and have done so since the nineteenth century when grain-

finished beef was considered a delicacy. Still, Americans were once addicted to canned vegetables and instant coffee. If the gourmet renaissance of the past decades has proved anything, it's that the human taste bud can be educated. We can learn to like flavor. We can change our mind-sets. Just like the cattle industry needs to do.

One of the most hopeful flickers for the future of cattle is coming out of Europe. Recognizing the carbon-reducing effects of grassland, the EU has started bankrolling "agrienvironmental" schemes, among which are grants to farmers for sucking carbon dioxide into their soil. In Europe, instead of subsidizing farmers to produce unnecessary food, the government is beginning to pay farmers to be environmental custodians. One such scheme involves reviving cattle breeds suited to actually living in the countryside. In Yorkshire, for instance, the "Limestone Country Project" pays farmers to plant wildflower meadows instead of annual grass fields. As poetic as these meadows appear to wistful tourists, they're not as productive as pure grass, so the cows that graze on them need to be hardier than the typical cows that end up in American feedlots. Braced by money from Brussels, farmers have reintroduced Belted Galloway cows and the glorious Highland cattle— all-terrain beeves that can survive a blizzard but that take a long time to grow to maturity (thirty long months for the Galloway).

The wildflower meadows are the stuff of Wordsworth, their flashes of crimson, sunburst, and white blending into the gentle violets of the hilltops. Underneath, the valleys of the Yorkshire Dales National Park are now speckled with beautiful, long-horned cattle, staring at hikers from under their woolly brows.

◆ Ethical Eating ◆

The King asked
The Queen and
The Queen asked

The Dairymaid:
"Could we have some butter for
The Royal slice of bread?"
The Queen asked
The Dairymaid,
The Dairymaid
Said, "Certainly,
I'll go and tell
The cow
Now
Before she goes to bed."

The Dairymaid
She curtsied,
And went and told
The Alderney:
"Don't forget the butter for
The Royal slice of bread."

The Alderney
Said sleepily:
"You'd better tell
His Majesty
That many people nowadays
Like marmalade
Instead."

—A. A. Milne, "The King's Breakfast"

In 1990, an environmental group called London Greenpeace (not the same as Greenpeace International), printed a leaflet entitled, "What's Wrong with McDonald's?" It made the now-familiar accusations of animal cruelty, deforestation, low wages, and childhood obesity, and the allegations were barbed enough to stick in the public mind.[24] McDonald's, fearing for its reputation as a kindly family business staffed by clowns, swatted two of the activists, Helen Steel and Dave Morris, with a megaton lawsuit. It became the longest-running libel trial in the history of the United Kingdom.

After about seven years and three hundred excruciating days in court, the Honorable Mr. Justice Bell declared that Steel and Morris had failed to prove their claims about ruined rain forests, heart disease and cancer, food poisoning, starvation in the Third World, and working conditions equivalent to an ungenerous sweatshop. He did, however, agree that the leaflet was accurate in claiming that McDonald's sold hamburgers to children by means of nefarious advertising. And it was responsible for cruelty to animals. The judge spoke sternly of imprisoned hens and wretched pigs, before addressing the future hamburgers themselves. He declared that although cattle may be frightened by the surroundings of the abattoir, and that some may be urged with electric prods, he did not find evidence that the animals waiting to be killed struggled, nor that they became "frantic as they watch the animal before them in the killing-line being prodded, beaten, electrocuted and knifed."

In this, the judge did not say that McDonald's is itself cruel to animals. He did say, however, that there is cruelty to animals inherent in some animal industry practices, and that the restaurant is "culpably responsible" for that cruelty in cases where it has close relationships with its suppliers. This close relationship would apply to slaughterhouses and egg farms, but not, say, to cow-calf ranches that are two steps removed from the fryer.

Although the ruling was a partial vindication of the beef industry, it did more to disgust the public than to assuage its fears, especially in Europe. Anyone who hadn't imagined the cows' ghastly troop onto the killing floor now had a fixed image of panicking steers, wide-eyed and rearing as they're pushed into abattoirs manned by the moral descendants of Auguste Pinochet. The fast-food business reeled under the bad press. Suddenly, public opinion held restaurateurs responsible for everything from fat children to the decline of the family farm. Protest campaigns sprouted like mushrooms in a cow pasture.[25]

Fast food, regardless of the realities of its business practices, is now forever equated with sadism, cancer, and an attitude toward labor best summed up by the words *Arbeit Macht Frei*. Documentary films and investigative books have fired a steady blast of best-selling broadsides against the industry. It's been a public relations debacle approaching the depths plumbed by tobacco or seal clubbing. You know you've got image problems when someone as institutionally muzzled as Prince Charles feels free, on a state visit to the United Arab Emirates in 2007, to suggest the idea of a government ban on McDonald's food.

The hamburger, and beef in general, is in need of good publicity. Ethical consumers—from sign-waving animal-rights activists, "ecosexual" yuppies, and parents puzzling over the malignancy of growth hormones—need reassurance, and the fast-food industry is trying to give it. Both McDonald's and Burger King now have "animal welfare advisory committees." In 2000, McDonald's told farmers that it required all of its meat suppliers to comply with new, ethical guidelines.[26] This includes inspections, restrictions on the use of electric prods, and standards for humanely stunning the animals before killing them. They also monitor how distressed the cattle behave, counting, for example, the number of cows that moo while awaiting slaughter. Burger King no longer buys meat from abattoirs in which animals are unable to walk to the killing floor, a measure designed to ensure that the cattle are transported in a manner that gives them, at least, a nod toward delicacy.[27]

So there's been progress. Consumers are beginning to aspire to an ideal of wholesomeness. There's a conception that something's amiss with meat, that things can be done better. The word *organic* is now a supermarket cliché. Even grocery stores in working-class neighborhoods sell "natural" sirloin strips at a steep markup over their unnatural cousins.

"The market [for natural beef] is still among a sophisticated consumer focused on other aspects than how cheaply he can fill his buggy at the supermarket," says Harris, the Tennessee cattleman. He sells much of his product at Whole Foods supermarkets, a chain of luxury grocery stores that's beyond the credit ratings of most Americans, but that glows with edible treasures. "It's a niche, but it's growing."

For two hundred years, economics has narrowed our focus onto the products we can take from cattle, and now we're beginning to discover that it pays to consider the animal's reputation as well. Ethical ice cream maker Ben and Jerry's is a lesson in the financial rewards of sustainable dairy farming.[28] Feel-good ice cream, "natural" steaks, and organic milk are symptoms of a slight, but significant, shift in the public eye that means that cattle are beginning to appear in a broader perspective. It's a start.

◆ Meden Agan ◆
Japanese Wagyu Beef

Leanness is no virtue in beef. Marbling—the degree to which meat is veined by white skeins of fat—is what gives beef its tenderness, basting the flesh in flavor as the grease melts during cooking. The Japanese have known this for centuries, but Americans are only beginning to overcome their twentieth-century disdain for the sensuous taste and visual purity of animal lard. We have a cultural preference for aged steak in which tenderness is brought on by decomposition. But no beef is sweeter, and more larded, than that of the Wagyu cow.

The Wagyu is the breed responsible for Kobe beef, a luxury meat that, like port wine or champagne, is named for its birthplace, in this case a Japanese shipping town on the western edge of the Osaka sprawl. The cows themselves are famous for living in indolence on quiet farms in the Hyogo Prefecture, eating buckets of high-calorie feed laced with tofu, drinking beer to stimulate their appetites, and being massaged with straw brushes. Stories abound about these bovine sybarites—the specialty diet, their alcohol rubs, their leisurely afternoon walks on the banks of the Miyagawa River, and their appalling cost of $300 per pound of raw meat. For a hundred years, these cows have been bred with the ideal of creating the perfectly marbled steak. This is beef as purest snobbery. Wagyu is the most elitist of meats in a country in which class consciousness runs in the tap water.

Looking at Wagyu beef as a lesson in animal welfare or environmental sustainability would be like looking at the wreck of the *Medusa* for tips on cruise ship protocol. In the name of marbling, the animals are fed a malnourishing diet that wracks them with illnesses.[29] Their lives are extraordinarily wasteful in grain and energy. But Wagyu has a lesson, not in farming, but in consumption. In the words that were carved above Apollo's temple at Delphi: *meden agan*. Nothing in excess.

The Japanese are not beef people. Like the Romans, they have always preferred the briny joys of fish. It was only after the Meiji Restoration of 1868 that meat was eaten at all—the twin threats of Buddhism and famine held such a grip on the islands that the flesh of four-legged animals had been banned from the cook pot for a thousand years. Animals were for pulling plows and for contemplating. Scores of generations of Japanese lived without ever having felt their mouths water at the smell of a grilled chop.

When Emperor Meiji did, finally, lift the ban, it was cosmopolitan Kobe that led the adoption of foreign eating habits. But even then, the Japanese never really took to eating the glistening wads of steak beloved by the West. They still ate their beef in slender, chopstick-friendly slices, used primarily as a garnish for rice and vegetables.

Although *Wa* means Japan, and *gyu* means beef, Wagyu cattle themselves are not truly native. In the nineteenth and early twentieth centuries, the government imported European breeds in bulk, breeding them into the native lines (very rare animals that are, oddly, genetically more akin to Europe's *Bos taurus* than to the *indicus* of Asia and the Philippines). By the end of the Second World War, four commercial Wagyu varieties had emerged, the most prominent of which is the Japanese Black.[30] This is a medium-sized meat cow with relatives among the Brown Swiss. She's useless for milking and she suffers calving problems due to thin pinbones, but her flesh is worthy of being carved into a pietà.

In a peculiar twist of history, the Japanese again closed their doors when, in the postwar period, the government tried to protect the domestic cattle industry by choking the export of Wagyu cattle. But as is so often the case in the looking-glass world of economics, it didn't work out as expected. A few cattle did leave the country, and, since the 1970s, several American and Australian farms have bred Wagyu. The astronomical costs of grain and farmland in Japan have created a huge Japanese market for these diaspora cows. Today, herds of Wagyu make a reverse crossing to the land of their ancestors. These imported Wagyu are promptly butchered, stamped with the label of Kobe beef, and then often mailed back to restaurants in Beverly Hills.

By the standards of resource conservation, the story of Kobe beef is atrocious. Intensive grain feeding, an unsparing investment of labor, and not one, but two trans-Pacific voyages. This is the stuff that leaves disciples of sustainable agriculture weeping into their oatmeal. It's clearly a useless model for large-scale cattle operations. And it wouldn't work if the Japanese, who buy nearly all the Wagyu beef on the market, demanded a full pound of flesh for their dinner.

The lesson of Wagyu is that there's a libertine's pleasure to be taken in this ivory, blood-jeweled meat, like cinnabar streaked with cream. Wagyu, clean of smoke and dressings, tastes more virginal than veal. It's beef before the Fall, and it costs a devil's ransom. That's what saves it. Wagyu, on account of its price, imposes restraint. There can be no Wagyu gorgers—no chicken-fried Wagyu booths in the county fair, no all-you-can-eat troughs at the Wagyu buffet, no triple-decker Wagyu burgers straining at the bun. This is beef that forces its consumer to compress his or her appetites, or learn to satiate them elsewhere.

The libertine, at least, knows this moral: Better a morsel of pleasure than a surfeit of junk. It's worth chewing over. And the lesson extends to beef in general.

"We shouldn't be eating gigantic plate-sized steaks," says Lauren Gwin of the U.S. Grassfed Association. "A big part of our sustainability problem is that we eat such vast quantities. If we cut our portion size slightly, the amount of beef we could produce in sustainable ways would be enough."

⌒⌒

CULINARY INTERLUDE

Wagyu Sashimi

Considering Wagyu's expense, you may as well plan a dinner of fried gold. But if your budget allows for a thick slab, sear the meat quickly in a hot pan or on a blazing grill, blackening it fast without allowing the inside to cook. Wagyu is ruined if the inner fat melts and drips away, or if heat burns off its perfume. To experience its subtle tangs and gelatinous, puddinglike texture, it should be eaten when it's quivering, velvety, and purple.

The most economical way to sample it is in the Japanese style—raw, and in very small portions:

Marinate the meat in equal parts premium soy sauce and dashi broth (the base for miso soup) for ten minutes, sprinkling chopped green onions into the bowl. Remove the meat and slice into strips about one-eighth of an inch thick. Arrange decorously and eat with chopsticks.

◆ Titus Salt, *the* Great Paternalist ◆

In the days before the city of Bradford turned into the municipal equivalent of a rotten lung, there lived a man named Titus Salt. He was a textile baron, but his mind wasn't solely steeped in ledger ink and dreams of profit. Like many other Victorians, he cultivated strong whiskers and Congregationalist morality, and he thought a great deal about Christian duty and the improvement of man, or at least of man's estate within this mortal coil.

Charles Dickens once called Bradford "the Beastliest of Places," and Salt vehemently agreed.[31] He looked out at the city's gusting soot, its smokestacks dribbling their fumes across canals black with excrement and cholera, and its clustered slums, rent apart by periodic bouts of disease only to rise again on a fresh raft of hungry bodies. He felt righteous umbrage. He also felt responsible. Salt had begun his career as a lowly wool stapler in his father's textile firm, but by midcentury he was the largest employer in a city that had mushroomed from 13,000 to 104,000 souls in fifty years. So it was a simple matter for him to get elected mayor of Bradford.

Salt ran his campaign on a platform of cleaning up the city's two-hundred-odd textile mills. He led by example. In his factories, he installed the finest nineteenth-century clean technology: tall smokestacks to disperse soot, and a contraption called the "Rodda Smoke Burner" that cut the filth spewed by furnaces. But the Bradford city councilmen were sluggish crusaders at best, and Salt abandoned politics in frustration, deciding to fulfill his ideals through the infinitely more efficient method of buying them. In 1853, on his fiftieth birthday, he unveiled what would be his life's great work.

Saltaire was its name. A model village built in the Aire Valley, about three miles from Bradford, Salt brought his workers to live there and work in his new mill, one that burned the cleanest fuels, spouted its smoke from the highest of smokestacks, and hid its machinery underground, to lessen the noise. As for the village, Salt's biographer, the Reverend R. Balgarnie, wrote in 1877:

> *[His vision] embraced what was still more dear to him,—the provision of comfortable dwellings, church, schools,—in fact, every institute which could improve the moral, mental and religious condition of the workpeople . . . in all there are twenty-two streets besides places, terraces, and roads, which contain 850 houses, and forty-five almshouses, making a total of 895 dwellings, covering an area of twenty five acres.[32]*

Not for nothing was Salt called "the great paternalist." He installed "watch towers" inside houses and workplaces, so he could spy on his employees, and he banned pubs, thinking them nests of political dissension. Utopia, thought Salt, was built on strict policing.

To celebrate his birthday and to formalize his stab at colonizing Yorkshire, Salt threw a big party. Balgarnie, who had a chronicler's love of enumeration, tells us that the menu included:

> Four hindquarters of beef, 40 chines of beef, 120 legs of mutton, 100 dishes of lamb, 40 hams, 40 tongues, 50 pigeon pies, 50 dishes of roast chicken, 20 dishes of roast duck, 30 braces of grouse, 30 braces of partridge, 50 dishes of potted meat, 320 plum puddings, 100 dishes of tartlets, 100 dishes of jellies.[33]

Two tons of meat were duly sliced, slopped out, and swallowed by his devoted, secretly monitored workers. Today, Salt's statue holds pride of place in Roberts Park, not far from the ornate cupola of Saltaire's Congregational Church, in which he is buried.

Saltaire, despite its hubristic name and its unsavory social engineering, was a tremendous success. Salt knew that a good business, one that looked to future profits as much as to the daily wool prices, depended on more than just financial margins. He needed a dependable workforce. And the workforce needed a dependable life. So he designed a town as a sustainable environment for the breeding and upkeep of late-nineteenth-century, lower-class Englishmen. That it was done out of enlightened self-interest is irrelevant, for it meant that his workers lived well, meaning they had superior food, housing, education, and work conditions when their peers in Bradford were choking in misery.

Saltaire weathered the death of both its founder and of the wool trade. When the mill closed, the village hunkered down to wait out a calamitous twentieth century. But unlike in other Yorkshire wool towns, the schools remained open, the terraced houses kept their doors painted and their yardwork neat. When the tourists arrived twenty years ago, Saltaire proved ready to meet the demand for curio shops, canal tours, and cappuccino. In 2001, the UN named it a World Heritage Sight. Saltaire, unlike the other neighborhoods of Bradford, survived.

The old Salts Mill hasn't churned out a textile in a hundred years, but it's not dormant. The approach is the same as it was in Salt's day—a descent from the street into a sunken court railed by black iron, cast in perpetual twilight by the mill itself, which is big. Battleship big. Glacier big. Or rather, it's as big as the vanished wealth and certitude of the Victorian Age. Inside, though, the hulk is alive, its rusting vitals ripped out and supplanted by an organic foods restaurant, a literary bookstore, and a surprisingly large collection of the works of celebrity artist David Hockney. The Olympian stone workfloors are now overseen by student waitresses, while California blues and Arizona reds shimmer and glow from canvases hung beneath ancient steam pipes, long since cooled.

Saltaire is alive today because it wasn't a slum, cobbled together on the cheap to gouge a quick rent out of drifting proles. It was built for human beings, using the needs of human beings as its blueprint. Then, when less stable communities fell apart, Saltaire had the resilience to survive until the economy clawed its way into a happier century.

When the cattle industry implodes, there may be a few Saltaires in the Wisconsin hills or on the Texas prairies. But most of the people whose lives depend on beef will, like Bradford's mill workers in the nineteenth century and its butchers in the twentieth, sink. It happens all the time. The history of economics is littered with wreckage. Industries capsize under nearsighted captains, or their bottoms fall out despite years of warning. Just ask a seventeenth-century Dutch tulip salesman, or a twentieth-century coal miner.

They say that King Solomon found a magic ring that had the power to make a sad man happy, and a happy man sad. It was a plain gold band inscribed with the words, "This too shall pass." Change is the only certainty, and, be it among Galapagos turtles or Wall Street financiers, adaptation is the only way to survive. Taking a page from Salt, the cattle industry is going to have to remember that cows, just like Victorian mill workers, aren't machines. They can't be forced into environments that treat them as such. Labor management practices have come a long way in a hundred years. It's time for animal husbandry to catch up.

There will have to be regulation. To the distaste of many a cowboy-hatted farmer, legislation will have to be passed and enforced, and government forms will need to be signed (but since most cowboy-hatted farmers are no strangers to government checks, their qualms shouldn't be too hard to swallow).

Wildflower meadows don't supplant grain fields unless there's a will for it. It will have to come from the industry. Beef barons will have to clamor and moo and send e-mails to their lobbyists. Government doesn't legislate wildflower meadows unless there's a will for it. As for the Great American Shopper, he or she will have to make a choice. Either walk the meat aisle with an eye for qualities like provenance, ecological impact, and sustainability, or look to canned beans.

∙ EPILOGUE ∙

There are many legends that tell of how the Masai came to exist. Some speak of an Israelite beginning and a long walk from the Red Sea. Others talk of a common father whose sons were like the branches of a mango tree. And others tell of how the people descended from heaven on a cowhide, arriving on Earth in the bleak Kerio Valley.

The valley was so hot and unwelcoming that the people's cows and children began dying of thirst. They needed to escape. As the elders gathered under a thorn tree to discuss the problem, they saw birds fluttering in the branches, building their nests out of fresh, green leaves. So the elders built a tall ladder for scouts to climb and watch the birds and to see where they had picked the shoots.

The scouts climbed up the ladder for days, until they arrived at a beautiful, verdant land. They collected green twigs to carry back and show the people where they had been, but when the people saw them, they grew cross.

"That's all very well," they said. "But how are we supposed to bring our cattle up the ladder to this green land? They can't very well climb, can they?"

So they built a great bridge out of the valley and up into the green land. But when half the people and half the cattle had crossed, the bridge gave way and collapsed, stranding the other half of the people behind in the desert.

The people who had made the crossing became the Masai, and those they abandoned in the parched valley were the Ilmek or "everyone else." This is how things came to be the way they are, how half of the people were left in the wilderness.

At the close of our carnivore dinner, we stared at the thickening grease on our plates and tried, very hard, to breathe. Then the waiters brought us a clod of cheesecake that we squinted at as if it were something unclean, like a dish of newts.

Gluttony is a capital sin, but unless they're felonies, sins aren't worth much anymore. Overeating is about as disgraceful as driving above the speed limit. And overeating, despite the 854 million hungry mouths in the world, isn't the real American vice.[1] One of the reasons for the rise of gourmet chic is that excessive pleasure in food, what Thomas Aquinas called *ardenter* (eagerness) and *studiose* (daintiness), is seen as a stamp of refinement. Even of intelligence. We feel no shame in relishing Pont L'Eveque above supermarket cheddar, despite what it may cost. The very sin that, in the fifteenth century, damned Dante's friend Ciacco to an afterlife of rotting in feculent mud has become a mark of good breeding.

To the religious, the price of gluttony isn't so much a bulbous midriff as a shrunken soul. Indulgence of the body means a neglect of the mind. If we meditate solely on our guts and glands and nerve endings, then these are the sum of our existence. The life of a paramecium is about as meaningful, and as large. But, then, we're biologically predisposed to gorge on hot dogs and chateaubriand alike—to scrounge for lipids, to glean every calorie out of a raw cow's hoof. Evolution has made eaters of us. It is our original sin.

Lolling under the weight of our dinner, we picked our teeth and talked about Kenya's tribal skirmishes in the 1990s, about the wickedness of politicians, and about that most chilling of problems, worse than any tick bite or mystery ulcer: the future.

"The youth aren't nostalgic," said Jerry. "They have their independence, so they don't think about the old ways. You know, I don't think that my children care about cattle."

It was true. One of Jerry's sons was entering business. Another wanted to study aeronautical engineering at MIT. Jerry's daughter was in boarding school, and would naturally dump her tribal connections at the first flash of city lights, choosing an office paycheck over marriage, cattle, and genital mutilation. Educated girls always did.

But Jerry still cared. That's why he drove around the countryside with a box of vaccination shots. It's why he drank chai with crotchety elders, coaxing them to sell their stock, crossbreed their herds, and maximize their land use; it's why he lost his temper with oafs in the Narok Town Council Slaughterhouse, and why he tossed wormy cow livers into the fire. And it's why, despite his pressed polo shirts, his home satellite dish, and his immaculate English syntax, Jerry was an unregenerate pastoralist. Like Charles Goodnight. Like Cuchulainn. Like Dumuzi and Abel. Like all the Masai since they had come down from heaven on their magic cowhide. Jerry's universe was defined by cattle—just as it had been when he was an adolescent squatting in a cave with a lump of bloody meat in his hand and a brainful of violent herbs. And, sitting under the air-conditioning with a glass of seltzer water and a winking cell phone, he knew that this part of his being, the broad plains under the herdsman's stars, was passing away.

A wild roar rose from the busload of wild Irish teenagers at the table next to us. They were red with drink, slopping their beers in their plates and mangling cigarettes with rubbery fingers. Swaying to their feet, they took snapshots of the Kenyan waiters, who grinned and lifted beef haunches for the camera. Trophies of crackling and flesh.

"Christ, I made a pig of meself!" laughed one of the kids. "I'll never eat a dinner like this again."

We paid the bill and walked out from under the electric sheen, into the darkness toward the hungry streets of Kibera.

⋄ ACKNOWLEDGMENTS ⋄

Many people need to be thanked for helping conceive, gestate, and deliver this book. Foremost are our families. We also wish to thank Jerry Ole Kina, our Masai hero; Cliff Moskow and Ledama Olekina at Maasai Education Discovery, and all the people of Masailand who gave us their friendship, help, and, most of all, trust.

Thanks to Jay Murray from Grill 23 in Boston for his steak expertise. Also to Pedro Trapote for showing us how fighting bulls are raised, and to Che Che Hirschfeld for his company, wit, and driving skills. We're indebted to Linda Luke from Luke & McKenna Inc. for allowing us to tap twenty-five years of cheese expertise, and to Alison and Colin Beaumont for sharing the intimacies of the lives of West Yorkshire butchers. Also to Carrie Balkom and Lauren Gwin of the American Grassfed Association, and to Will Harris of White Oaks Pastures.

Thanks and love to family members for providing unvarnished opinions and unflinching support, namely Dr. David Fraser (the elder); Mrs. Nancy Fraser; Elizabeth and Chris Fraser; also to Ramune Rimas and Paul Rimas for encouragement and sustenance. Immeasurable thanks to our wives, Laura Bravo and Christine de Vuono, for their patience and reading. Also an extra big thank-you to Laura for translating.

More thanks to Michael Blanding, for helping us find an agent, and to Larry Weissman, for being the agent who took a pair of untested writers under his wing. Thanks to David Highfill, our editor, and Gabe Robinson at William Morrow for helpful guidance and comments all along.

Many thanks to George and Christian for the game.

For recipe-testing, we're indebted to Nick Altschuller, Rich Levine, and Megan Lisagor at *The Improper Bostonian*.

Our utmost gratitude to Mike Smith for being generous with his ideas on the origins of Hebrew monotheism. And to various members of the Sustainability Research Institute, School of Earth and Environment, University of Leeds, for thought-provoking discussions, and for indulging more conversations on cows than they might have liked.

We would have been adrift in the UK landscape without the kind and enthusiastic assistance of Miles Johnson from the Yorkshire Dales National Park. In addition, aspects of this book were inspired by results that have emerged through an academic research project funded through the "Rural Economy and Land Use Programme." The Rural Economy and Land Use Programme is funded jointly by the United Kingdom's Economic and Social Research Council, the Biotechnology and Biological Sciences Research Council, and the Natural Environment Research Council, with additional funding from the Department for Environment, Food and Rural Affairs and the Scottish Executive Environment and Rural Affairs Department. In particular, the members of the "sustainable uplands" at the Universities of Leeds provided endless discussions on the role of animal grazing in the hills of Northern England.

And, of course, thanks to the members of the *Bos genus* and the people who raise them—past, present, and future.

Again, our gratitude and love to our wives Laura Bravo and Christine de Vuono. All is for you.

⋆ ENDNOTES ⋆

CHAPTER 1

1. C. Gottlieb, "The Meaning of Bull and Horse in *Guernica*," *Art Journal* 24 (1964–65): 106–112. The quote is on p. 109.

2. Ibid.

3. W. Proweller, "Picasso's 'Guernica': A Study in Visual Metaphor," *Art Journal* 30 (1971): 240–248.

4. D. Schneider, "The Painting of Pablo Picasso: A Psychoanalytic Study," *College Art Journal* 7 (1947–48): 81–95.

5. J. M. De Cossio, *Los Toros* (Madrid: Espasa-Calpe, 1943).

6. *King James Bible*, Reference edition.

7. C. Wood and C. Knipmeyer, "Global Climate Change and Environmental Stewardship by Ruminant Livestock Producers," *Applied Environmental Science: Student Reference*, USEPA, NCAE, and FFA Foundation, 1998.

8. J. Berger, "Predator Harassment as a Defensive Strategy in Ungulates," *American Midland Naturalist* 102 (1979): 197–199.

9. G. Page, "Raptor Predation on Wintering Shorebirds," *The Condor* 77 (1975): 73–83.

10. M. Ruspoli, *The Cave of Lascaux: The Final Photographs* (New York: Harry N. Abrams, 1987).

11. T. Van Vuure, "History, Morphology and Ecology of the Aurochs (*Bos Primigenius*)," *Lutra* 45 (2002): 3–17.

12. J. Caesar, *The Gallic Wars*, trans. W. A. McDevitte (1868), http://classics

.mit.edu/Caesar/gallic.html (accessed May 24, 2007). The quote is found in section 6.28.

13. J. Dunn, trans., *Táin bó Cúailnge* (London: David Nutt Publishers, 1914). The quote is in section 29.

14. T. Dewey and J. Ng, *Bos taurus. Animal Diversity Web,* 2001, http://animaldiversity.ummz.umich.edu/site/accounts/information/Bos_taurus.html (accessed March 19, 2007).

15. S. Budiansky, *The Covenant of the Wild: Why Animals Chose Domestication* (New Haven, CT: Yale University Press, 1999). See also S. Gould, *The Panda's Thumb: More Reflections on Natural History* (New York: Norton, 1980).

16. Van Vuure, "The History, Morphology and Ecology of the Aurochs," 4.

17. R. O'Connell, *Ride of the Second Horseman: The Birth and Death of War* (Oxford and New York: Oxford University Press, 1995).

18. Ibid., 57.

19. O'Connell, *Ride of the Second Horseman.*

20. F. Gasse, "Hydrological Changes in the African Tropics Since the Last Glacial Maximum," *Quaternary Science Reviews* 19 (2000): 189–211.

21. A. Smith, "Review Article: Cattle Domestication in North Africa," *The African Archaeological Review* 4 (1986): 197–203.

22. N. Wade, "Lactose Tolerance in East Africa Points to Recent Evolution," *New York Times,* December 11, 2006.

23. Ibid.

24. A. Sherratt, "Animal Traction and the Transformation of Europe (English translation)," in *Proceedings of the Frasnois Conference,* ed. P. Pétrequin, 2005. English version available at http://www.archatlas.dept.shef.ac.uk/people/Frasnois.pdf (accessed May 25, 2007).

25. O'Connell, *Ride of the Second Horseman.*

26. G. Leick, *A Dictionary of Ancient Near Eastern Mythology* (London: Routledge, 1991).

27. T. Jacobsen, *The Treasures of Darkness: A History of Mesopotamian Religion* (New Haven, CT: Yale University Press, 1978).

28. D. Wolkstein, *Inanna* (New York: Harper Perennial, 1983).

29. E. Hemingway, *Death in the Afternoon* (New York: Vintage, 2000). The quote is on page 64.

30. Ibid., 4.

31. Translation by Laura Bravo.

32. J. de la Cal, "El toro no es tradicion, es negocio," *El Mundo*, December 24, 2006.

CHAPTER 2

1. A. Bowman, *Life and Letters on the Roman Frontier: Vindolanda and Its People*, 2nd ed. (London: British Museum Press, 2004).

2. R. L. Beck, "Entry on Mithras," in *The Oxford Classical Dictionary*, eds. S. Hornblower and A. Spawforth (London: Oxford University Press, 2003).

3. Pliny the Elder, *Natural History*, trans. J. Healy (New York: Penguin, 1991). The quote is on p. 183.

4. Apicius, *Apicii librorum x qui dicuntur de re coquinaria quae extant*, trans. Louise Hope, Ted Garvin, David Starner, and the Online Distributed Proofreading Team at http://www.pgdp.net (Project Gutenberg, 1922 imprint), http://www.gutenberg.org/etext/16439 (accessed June 28, 2007). The quote comes from Book II, 53.

5. M. Balter, *The Goddess and the Bull: Catalhoyuk—An Archaeological Journey to the Dawn of Civilization* (New York: Simon & Schuster, 2005).

6. Ibid.

7. Ibid.

8. Ibid., 177.

9. Homer, *The Odyssey*, trans. S. Butcher. (London: Macmillan and Co., 1885), posted on classcs.mit.edu/Homer/odyssey.12.xii.html.

10. Anonymous. *The Epic of Gilgamesh*, trans. N. Sandars. (New York: Penguin, 2007). The quote is on page 97.

11. Ovid, *Metamorphoses*, trans. S. Garth, J. Dryden, A. Pope, J. Addison, and W. Congreve, 1717.

12. Anonymous, "Entry on Mithras," in *The Oxford Classical Dictionary*, eds. S. Hornblower and A. Spawforth (London: Oxford University Press, 2003).

13. K. Armstrong, *A Short History of Myth* (Edinburgh: Canongate, 2005).

14. R. Ackerman, *J. G. Frazer: His Life and Work* (Cambridge: Cambridge University Press, 1987).

15. Ibid.

16. J. Frazer, *The Golden Bough* (London: Oxford University Press, 1998), section 7.5.

17. R. Graves, *Larousse Encyclopedia of Mythology* (London: Paul Hamlyn, 1960).

18. L. De Heusch, "The Symbolic Mechanisms of Sacred Kingship: Rediscovering Frazer," *Journal of the Royal Anthropological Institute* 3 (1997): 213–232.

19. Ibid., 219.

20. F. R. Walton and J. Scheid, "Entry on Cybele," in *The Oxford Classical Dictionary*, eds. S. Hornblower and A. Spawforth (London: Oxford University Press, 2003).

21. Herodotus, *The History*, trans. D. Grene (Chicago, University of Chicago Press, 1987), section 3.28.

22. W. Burkert, *Greek Religion: Archaic and Classical* (Oxford: Blackwell Publishers, 1987).

23. D. Wengrow, *The Archaeology of Early Egypt. Social Transformations in North-East Africa, 10,000–2,650 B.C.* (Cambridge: Cambridge World Archaeology Series, Cambridge University Press, 2006).

24. Ibid., 95.

25. Wengrow, *Archaeology of Early Egypt.*

26. M. Harris, *Cows, Pigs, Wars, and Witches* (New York: Vintage Paperbacks, 1989), 18.

27. Food and Agriculture Organziation of the United Nations, FAOSTAT, Rome, UN, 2007, http://faostat.fao.org/ (accessed September 18, 2007).

28. Anonymous, *A Beef with India*, Compassion Over Killing Web Page, 2004, http://www.cok.net/camp/writers/04/1116-sa.php (accessed July 8, 2007).

29. M. Smith, *The Origins of Biblical Monotheism: Israel's Polytheistic Background and the Ugaritic Texts* (Oxford: Oxford University Press, 2001).

30. Ibid. Smith notes Genesis 49 and Psalm 82 as examples.

31. Ibid.

32. Ibid.

CHAPTER 3

1. M. Gimbutas, *The Balts* (London: Praeger, 1963/1968).

2. T. Kinsella, trans., *The Tain* (Oxford: Oxford University Press, 2002), 91–92.

3. T. Kinsella, "Introduction," *The Tain* (Oxford: Oxford University Press, 2002).

4. Kinsella, *The Tain*.

5. Ibid., 192.

6. R. O'Connell, *Ride of the Second Horseman: The Birth and Death of War* (Oxford and New York: Oxford University Press, 1997).

7. A. Leahy, *Heroic Romances of Ireland* (London: David Nutt, 1906).

8. Full texts of both poems are at www.sacred-texts.com/neu/hroi/hroiv2.htm.

9. Ibid.

10. K. Armstrong, *The Great Transformation: The World in the Time of Buddha, Socrates, Confucius and Jeremiah* (New York: Knopf, 2006).

11. R. Linton, "Nomad Raids and Fortified Pueblos," *American Antiquity* 10 (1944): 28–32.

12. O'Connell, *Ride of the Second Horseman*.

13. Tacitus, *The Agricola and the Germania,* trans. H. Mattingly and S. A. Handford (London: Penguin, 1970), section 14.

14. Ibid.

15. R. Manning, *Swordsmen: The Martial Ethos in the Three Kingdoms* (London: Oxford University Press, 2003).

16. T. Gomi, "On Dairy Productivity at Ur in the Late Ur iii Period," *Journal of the Economic and Social History of the Orient* 23 (1980): 1–42.

17. 1 Samuel 17:18.

18. M. Wolfsperger, "Trace-Element Analysis of Medieval and Early-Modern Skeletal Remains from Western Austria for Reconstruction of Diet," *Homo* 43 (1993): 278–294.

19. Note: the authors have not tried these recipes, but have gleaned this information from a range of sources including: B. Ciletti, *Making Great Cheese* (Lark Books, Asheville, NC, 1999), 88–89, http://www.gourmetsleuth.com/recipe_cheddarcheese.htm and http://www.allotment.org.uk/allotment_foods/3_Making_Cheddar_Cheese.php.

20. New Advent, *The Catholic Encyclopedia*, 2007, http://www.newadvent.org/cathen/index.html (accessed July 27, 2007).

21. Bede, *The Lives of the Holy Abbots of Weremouth and Jarrow Benedict,*

Ceolfrid, Easterwine, Sigfrid, and Huetberht, circa 716, trans. J. Giles in *The Medieval Sourcebook,* http://www.fordham.edu/halsall/basis/bede-jarrow .html (accessed July 15, 2007).

22. R. Sullivan, "The Carolingian Missionary and the Pagan," *Speculum* 28 (1953): 705–740.

23. The quote is from the monastic code called "rule of the master" that was similar to the Benedictine Rule, dating to the sixth century. This is quoted in D. Bazell, "Strive Amongst the Table Fellows," *Journal of the American Academy of Religion* 65 (1997): 73–99.

24. K. Pearson, "Nutrition and the Early Medieval Diet," *Speculum* 72 (1997): 1–32.

25. K. Ambrose, "A Medieval Food List from the Monastery of Cluny," *Gastronomica* 6 (2006): 14–20.

26. Thanks to Linda Luke of Luke-McKenna for help in compiling this list. Additional references are taken from R. Scott, *Cheesemaking Practice* (London: Applied Science Publishers Ltd., 1981). Also, thanks to the Lawsons at the Skipton town market for their help in ordering a real Muenster.

27. S. Mennell, *All Manners of Food* (Oxford: Basic Blackwell, 1985).

28. Medieval Cookery, "Medieval Cookery–Cook Book Analysis," www .medievalcookery.com/stats/stats.shtm (accessed May 15, 2006).

29. This translation can be found at http://www.godecookery.com/ alabama/alabam02.html#stw (accessed February 14, 2007).

30. J. Oliver, *A Source Book for Medieval History* (New York: Scribner's, 1905).

31. G. Fraser, *The Steel Bonnets: The Story of the Anglo-Scottish Border Reivers* (London: Barrie and Jenkins, 1971).

CHAPTER 4

1. J. De Vries, "The Role of the Rural Sector in the Development of the Dutch Rural Economy: 1500–1700," *Journal of Economic History* 31 (1971): 266–268.

2. S. Hartlib, *The Compleat Husband-Man: Or, A Discourse of the Whole Art of Husbandry; Both Forraign and Domestick* (London: Edward Brewster at the Crane in Paul's Church-yard, 1659).

3. G. Fussell, "Low Countries' Influence on English Farming," *English Historical Review* 74 (1959): 611–622.

4. Hartlib, *The Compleat Husband-Man,* 38.

5. Ibid, 38.

6. Quoted in M. Syvret and J. Stevens, *Balleine's History of Jersey* (Chichester: Phillimore, 1981).

7. A. S. Truswell, "The a2 Milk Case: A Critical Review," *European Journal of Clinical Nutrition* 59 (2004): 623.

8. Fairbrae Farm, "What Is a2 Milk?", 2007, http://www.fairbraemilk.com/atwomilk.htm (accessed January 16, 2007).

9. D. Piper, "Gainsborough at the Tate Gallery," *The Burlington Magazine* 95 (1953): 245–247.

10. H. Pawson, *Robert Bakewell, Pioneer Livestock Breeder* (London: C. Lockwood & Son, 1957).

11. P. Stanley, *Robert Bakewell and the Longhorn Breed of Cattle* (Ipswich: Farming Press, 1995).

12. J. Gribbin, *Science: A History* (London: Penguin, 2003).

13. W. Hazlitt, *Old Cookery Books and Ancient Cuisine* (London: Popular Edition, 1902).

14. Stanley, *Robert Bakewell and the Longhorn Breed of Cattle.*

15. P. Boden, "The Limestone Quarrying Industry of North Derbyshire," *The Geographical Journal* 129 (1960): 53–62.

16. Stanley, *Robert Bakewell and the Longhorn Breed of Cattle.*

17. Ibid.

18. Limestone Country Project Web Site, 2007, http://www.limestonecountry.org.uk/NetBuildPro/process/11/contactUs.html (accessed July 26, 2007).

19. Stanley, *Robert Bakewell and the Longhorn Breed of Cattle.*

20. D. Chipman, "New Light on the Career of Nuño Beltran de Guzman," *The Americas* 19 (1963), 341–348.

21. L. Simpson, *Many Mexicos* (Berkeley: University of California Press, 1960), 33–34.

22. P. De Fuentes, *The Conquistadores: First-Person Accounts of the Conquest of Mexico* (London: University of Oklahoma Press, 1993). The quote is on page 199.

23. Ibid., 243, n. 4.

24. D. Chipman, "The Traffic in Indian Slaves in the Province of Pánuco, New Spain, 1523–1533," *The Americas* 23 (1966): 142–155.

25. De Fuentes, *The Conquistadores.* The quote is on page 298.

26. Chipman, "The Traffic in Indian Slaves."

27. S. Trifilo, "The Gaucho: His Changing Image," *Pacific Historic Review* 33 (1964): 395–403.

28. E. Tinker, "The Horsemen of the Americas," *Hispanic American Historical Review* 42 (1962): 191–198. The quote is on p. 192.

29. Ibid.

30. K. Butzer, "Cattle and Sheep from Old to New Spain: Historical Antecedents," *Annals of the Association of American Geographers* 78 (1988): 29–56.

31. Ibid.

32. C. Bishko, "The Peninsular Background of Latin American Cattle Ranching," *Hispanic American Historical Review* 32 (1952): 491–515.

33. Butzer, "Cattle and Sheep from Old to New Spain."

34. W. Doolittle, "Las Marismas to Pánuco to Texas: The Transfer of Open Range Cattle Ranching from Iberia Through Northeast Mexico," *Yearbook, Conference of Latin Americanist Geographers* 13 (1987): 3–11.

35. Bishko, "The Peninsular Background of Latin American Cattle Ranching," 498.

36. A. Sluyter, "The Ecological Origins and Consequences of Cattle Ranching in Sixteenth-Century New Spain," *Geographical Review* 86 (1996): 161–177. The quote is on p. 168.

37. Doolittle, "Las Marismas to Pánuco to Texas."

38. E. Fratkin, "East African Pastoralism in Transition: Maasai, Boran, and Rendille Cases," *African Studies Review* 44 (2001): 1–25.

CHAPTER 5

1. D. Sinor, "The Mongols in the West," *Journal of Asian History* 33 (1999): 1–44.

2. C. Spinage, *Cattle Plague: A History* (New York: Kluwer Academic, 2003).

3. Ibid.

4. World Organization for Animal Health (OIE), "Animal Disease Data:

Rinderpest," Paris, OIE, 2002, http://www.oie.int/eng/maladies/fiches/a_
A040.htm (accessed August 15, 2007).

5. Commissioners Appointed to Inquire into the Origin and Nature of the
Cattle Plague, *Third Report,* London, 1866, presented to both Houses of Parliament by Command of Her Majesty. The quote comes from Part I, "Symptoms."

6. J. Kastner and D. Powell, "The SPS Agreement: Addressing Historical
Factors in Trade Dispute Resolution," *Agriculture and Human Values* 19
(2002): 283–292.

7. J. Fisher, "Cattle Plagues Past and Present," *Journal of Contemporary
History* 32 (1998): 215–228.

8. Quoted in Spinage, *Cattle Plague.* The quote is on page 5.

9. M. Worboys, "Germ Theory of Disease and British Veterinary Medicine, 1860–1890," *Medical History* 35 (1991): 308–327.

10. Commissioners Appointed to Inquire into the Origin and Nature of
the Cattle Plague, *Third Report,* London, 1866, presented to both Houses of
Parliament by Command of Her Majesty.

11. Spinage, *Cattle Plague,* 498.

12. Spinage, *Cattle Plague,* 502.

13. Spinage, *Cattle Plague.* The quote is on page 525.

14. H. Prins and V. D. Jeugd, "Herbivore Population Crashes and Wood-
land Structure in East Africa," *Journal of Ecology* 81 (1993): 305–314.

15. Fonck, 1894, quoted in Spinage, *Cattle Plague.* The quote is on
page 639.

16. World Organization for Animal Health (OIE), "Short History of the
OIE," Paris, OIE, 2002, http://www.oie.int/eng/OIE/en_histoire.htm?e1d1
(accessed August 15, 2007).

17. Food and Agriculture Organization of the United Nations, FAOSTAT,
Rome, FAO, 2007, http://faostat.fao.org/ (accessed September 17, 2007).

18. We are indebted to Mr. Miles Johnson, archaeologist at the Yorkshire
Dales National Park, for his time and enthusiasm in helping with the research
for this section.

19. J. Herriot, *The Best of James Herriot* (New York: St. Martin's Press,
1982). The quote is on pages 11 and 24.

20. World Holstein-Friesian Federation, Statistics, 2006, http://www.whff
.info/index.php?content=statistics& (accessed July 15, 2007).

21. M. Godbout, "Researchers from the Université de Montréal Faculty of Veterinary Medecine and l'Alliance Boviteq succeeded in cloning Starbuck," University of Montreal Press Release, 2000, http://www.iforum.umontreal .ca/Communiques/ArchivesCommuniques/2000/200920_ang.htm (accessed July 14, 2007).

22. Centre d'insémination artificielle du Québec, Web page on breeding cow called Starbuck, 2007, http://www.ciaq.com/Estarb2.htm#ancre2 (accessed July 14, 2007).

23. R. Mitchell, "The First Modern War, R.I.P.," *Reviews in American History* 17 (1989): 552–558.

24. D. Sponenberg and T. Olson, "Colonial Spanish Cattle in the USA: History and Present Status," *Archivos de Zootecnia* 41 (1992): 401–414.

25. J. Dobie, *The Longhorns* (Boston: Little Brown & Co., 1941).

26. A. Halloran and C. Shrader, "Longhorn Cattle Management on Wichita Mountains Wildlife Refuge," *Journal of Wildlife Management* 24 (1960): 191–196.

27. T. Haygood, "Texas Fever," *Handbook of Texas Online,* University of Texas, 2007, http://www.tsha.utexas.edu/handbook/online/articles/TT/awt1 .html (accessed April 12, 2007).

28. T. Jordan, "The Origin of Anglo-American Cattle Ranching in Texas: A Documentation of Diffusion from the Lower South," *Economic Geography* 45 (1969): 63–87.

29. J. Otto and N. Anderson, "Cattle Ranching in the Venezuelan Llanos and the Florida Flatwoods: A Problem in Comparative History," *Comparative Studies in Society and History* 28 (1986): 672–683.

30. J. Didion, *Slouching Towards Bethlehem* (New York: Washington Square Press, 1968). The quote is on pages 44–45.

31. G. Autry, *Gene Autry's Cowboy Code,* http://www.geneautry.com/ geneautry/geneautry_cowboycode.html (accessed August 28, 2007).

32. R. Brown, "Western Violence: Structure, Values, Myth," *The Western Historical Quarterly* 24 (1993): 4–20. The quote is on page 15.

33. H. Anderson, "Goodnight, Charles," *The Handbook of Texas,* 2002, http://www.tsha.utexas.edu/handbook/online/articles/GG/fgo11.html (accessed April 12, 2007).

34. A. Graybill, "Rural Police and the Defense of the Cattleman's Empire in Texas and Alberta, 1875–1900," *Agricultural History* 79 (2005): 253–280.

35. H. Brayer, "The Influence of British Capital on the Western Range-Cattle Industry," *Journal of Economic History* 9 (1949): 85–98.

36. D. Galenson, "The End of the Chisholm Trail," *Journal of Economic History* 34 (1974): 350–364.

37. E. Dale, "The Cow Country in Transition," *Mississippi Valley Historical Review* 24 (1937): 3–20. The quote is on pages 7 and 8.

38. W. Webb, *The Great Plains* (Waltham, MA: Ginn and Company, 1931).

39. R. Dykstra, *The Cattle Towns* (Lincoln: University of Nebraska Press, 1968).

40. C. Hutson, "Texas Fever in Kansas, 1866–1930," *Agricultural History* 68 (1994): 74–104. The quote is on page 81.

41. Hutson, "Texas Fever in Kansas, 1866–1930," 80.

42. M. Welch, "The Spanish Fever: How They Treat Texas Cattle on the Border," *Prairie Farmer* 39 (1868), 98.

43. Hutson, "Texas Fever in Kansas."

44. R. Dennen, "Cattle Trailing in the Nineteenth Century," *Journal of Economic History* 35 (1975): 458–460.

45. Devil's Rope Museum, "A Brief History of Barbed Wire," Devil's Rope Museum, McLean Texas, 2007, http://www.barbwiremuseum.com/index.htm (accessed August 14, 2007).

46. J. McFadden, "Monopoly in Barbed Wire: The Formation of the American Steel and Wire Company," *The Business History Review* 52 (1978): 465–489.

47. Texas Beef Council, Beef Recipes, 2007, http://www.txbeef.org/recipe.php3?944688139 (accessed July 16, 2007).

48. A. Davidson, *Oxford Companion to Food* (Oxford: Oxford University Press, 1999).

49. J. Williams, *Wagonwheel Kitchens: Food on the Oregon Trail* (Lawrence: University of Kansas Press, 1993).

50. M. Marchello and J. Garden-Robinson, "Jerky Making: Then and Now, *North Dakota State University's College of Agriculture, Food Systems and Natural Resources,* 1999, http://www.ag.ndsu.edu/pubs/yf/foods/fn580w.htm (accessed August 14, 2007).

51. The Chicago Historical Society's Homepage, *The Birth of the Chicago Union Stock Yards,* 2001, http://www.chicagohs.org/history/stockyard/stock1.html (accessed August 31, 2007).

52. U. Sinclair, *The Jungle* (New York: Penguin, 1985). The quote is on page 98.

53. Ibid., 120.

54. For a discussion on the origins of this poem, see *Cowboy Poetry,* 2007, http://www.cowboypoetry.com/whoknows4.htm#Longhorn (accessed July 16, 2007).

CHAPTER 6

1. Three Dales Quality Local Meat Web Page, http://www.threedales.co .uk/index.php (accessed May 31, 2007).

2. Meat Info, online Meat Trades Journal, 2007, http://www.meatinfo .co.uk/ (accessed, March 15, 2007).

3. Osborn Samuel Gallery, *Biography of Peter Kinley,* 2007, http:// osbornesamuel.com/pages/biography/41088.html (accessed March 15, 2007).

4. J. Clay, *World Agriculture and the Environment* (Washington, DC: Island Press, 2004).

5. National Agricultural Statistics Service, "All Cattle & Beef Cows: Number of Operations by Year, US," http://www.nass.usda.gov/Charts_and_ Maps/Cattle/acbc_ops.asp (accessed March 16, 2007).

6. For a review of popular works on this subject, please see J. Rifkin, *Beyond Beef* (New York: Plume, 1993); A. Kimbrell, ed., *The Fatal Harvest Reader: The Tragedy of Industrial Agriculture* (Washington, DC: Island Press, 2002); E. Schlosser, *Fast Food Nation* (London: Allen Lane, 2001).

7. Metropolitan Museum of Art, Details on John Curry, Collection Highlights, http://www.metmuseum.org/Works_of_Art/viewOne.asp?dep=21& viewmode=0&item=42.154 (accessed March 16, 2007).

8. U.S. Department of Agriculture, "Changes in Size and Location of U.S. Dairy Farms," in *Profits, Costs, and the Changing Structure of Dairy Farming /* ERR-47 Economic Research Service, USDA, 2006.

9. D. Jackson-Smith and B. Barham, "Dynamics of Dairy Industry Restructuring in Wisconsin," in *Dairy Industry Restructuring: Research in Rural Sociology and Development,* vol. 8, eds. H. Schwarzweller and A. Davidson (Amsterdam: JAI, 2000). Please see page 115.

10. R. Knutson and R. Loyns, "Understanding Canadian/United States Dairy Disputes," in *Proceedings of the Second Annual Canada/U.S. Agricultural*

and Food Policy Systems Information Workshop, eds. R. Knutson and R. Loyns (Guelph, Canada: University of Guelph, 1996).

11. W. Butler and C. Wolf, "California Dairy Production: Unique Policies and Natural Advantages," in *Dairy Industry Restructuring: Research in Rural Sociology and Development,* vol. 8, eds. H. Schwarzweller and A. Davidson (Amsterdam: JAI, 2000).

12. Food and Agriculture Association, *Livestock's Long Shadow* (Rome: United Nations, 2006).

13. A. Hovey, "Nebraska Hog, Cattle Farmers Take Losses as Grain Prices Soar," *Lincoln Journal Star,* May 2, 2008, http://www.siouxcityjournal.com/articles/2008/04/13/news/latest_news/doc4802161024de8996013082.txt (accessed May 2, 2008).

14. J. Steinbeck, *The Grapes of Wrath* (New York: Penguin, 2002).

15. J. Lawrence, "Impact of Higher Corn Prices on Feed Costs," *Iowa Farm Outlook,* October 1–2, 2006.

16. W. E. Riebsame, S. A. Changnon, and T. R. Karl. *Drought and Natural Resource Management in the United States* (Boulder, CO: Westview Press, 1991).

17. K. R. Laird, S. C. Fritz, K. A. Maasch, and B. F. Cumming, "Greater Drought Intensity and Frequency Before A.D. 1200 in the Northern Great Plains, U.S.A," *Nature* 384 (1996): 552–554.

18. N. Rosenberg, D. Epstein, D. Wang, L. Vail, R. Srinivasan, and J. Arnold, "Possible Impacts of Global Warming on the Hydrology of the Ogallala Aquifer Region," *Climatic Change* 42 (1999): 677–692.

19. Texas Water Development Board, *Surveys of Irrigation in Texas 1958, 1964, 1969, 1974, 1979, 1984, 1989, and 1994.* Report no. 347. (Austin: Texas Water Development Board, 1996).

20. B. Terrell, P. N. Johnson, and E. Segarra, "Ogallala Aquifer Depletion: Economic Impact on the Texas High Plains," *Water Policy* (2002), 4, 33–46.

21. E. Lambin, B. Turner, H. Geist, S. Agbola, A. Angelsen, J. Bruce, O. Coomes, et al., "The Causes of Land-Use and Land-Cover Change: Moving Beyond the Myths," *Global Environmental Change* 11 (2001): 261–269.

22. Food and Agriculture Association, *Livestock's Long Shadow.*

23. Interview with Lauren Gwin, December 31, 2007.

24. Mcspotlight, *The Mclibel Story,* 2007, http://www.mcspotlight.org (accessed March 15, 2007).

25. S. Gifford, *PETA's Letter to Safeway Explaining That the Decision to Treat Animals with Basic Decency Is Up to Safeway*, 2001, http://www.goveg.com/shameway_let9-14.asp (accessed March 15, 2007).

26. H. Mayer, *Animal Welfare Verification in Canada*, Canadian Council of Grocery Distributors, 2002, http://www.facs.sk.ca/pdf/other/animal_welfare_verification_Canada.pdf (accessed March 15, 2007).

27. Canadian Federation of Humane Societies, "McDonald's and Burger King Leading the Way," 2002, http://cfhs.ca/info/mcdonald%E2_s_and_burger_king_leading_the_way/ (accessed March 15, 2007).

28. C. Bylin, R. Misra, M. Murch, and W. Rigterink, *Sustainable Agriculture: An On-Farm Assessment Tool* (Ann Arbor, MI: University of Michigan, 2004).

29. H. Kawachi, "Micronutrients Affecting Adipogenesis in Beef Cattle," *Animal Science Journal* 77 (2006): 463–471.

30. J. Longworth, *Beef in Japan* (Brisbane: University of Queensland Press, 1983).

31. J. Reynolds, *The Great Paternalist* (London: Maurice Temple Smith, 1983). The quote is on page 89.

32. R. Balgarnie, *Sir Titus Salt, Baronet* (Settle, Yorkshire: Brenton Publishing, 1877). The quote is on page 135.

33. Ibid., 38.

EPILOGUE

1. Food and Agriculture Organization of the United Nations, *State of Food Insecurity in the World 2006* (Rome: FAO, 2006).

· INDEX ·

Book of Ezekiel, 48
Book of Genesis, 24, 185
Cain and Abel, 28
*The Birth of the Gods and the Origins
   of Agriculture* (Cauvin), 52
bison, 14
blood, symbolism of, 63–64
Bonilla, Adolfo de, 30
Book of the Dun Cow, 81
Border Reivers, 95–98
Bos indicus, 21
Bos primigenius, 16–20, 21, 155
Bos taurus, 21
Bos taurus ibericus, 128
bovid family, 21
bovinae, 21
bovine babesiosis, 155
bovine pleuropneumonia, 134
Bradford, West Yorkshire, 175–76,
   204–5
Brahman cows of India, 66–67
Breuil, Abbè Henri, 17
Brie cheese, 91
brisket, 15
British Navy, 116
Brown Bull of Cuailnge, 19, 78
Bucolics (Virgil), 60
Budiansky, Stephen, 22
bullfighting, 6–9, 29–38
bulls
   bucking bulls, 168
   Bull El, 69–70
   and bullfighting, 6–9, 29–38
   bull-leaping ritual, 59–60
   Bull of Heaven, 28, 56–57
   bull riding, 167–68
   Egyptian worship of, 64–66
   running of the bulls, 8–9
   sacred image of, 48, 69–70
   sacrificed to the gods, 46, 63–64
   tail meat of, 37–38

Burchell, John, 143
Burger King, 200
butchers, 135, 145, 171, 176–78
butter, 152

C

Caesar, Julius, 19
calves, golden, 68–69
Cambyses, King of Persia, 64–65
Camembert cheese, 91
carbon dioxide, 194, 197
Çatalhöyük, 49–53
cattle. *See also* cattle raids
   bride-price paid by, 80, 101
   Cattle of the Sun legend, 53–55
   drives, 158–61
   herds, 13–14, 27
   Latin word for, 75
   Masai, crossbreeding of, 137
   Mexican, 122–26
   origins of word, 84
   ranching, 122–26, 122–30
   sacrificed to the gods, 53–55
   Spanish, 122–30
cattle raids
   Border Reivers, 95–98
   Masai, 39–42, 98–101
   medieval, 79–84, 95, 127
cattle traders, 172
Cauvin, Jacques, 52
Charlemagne, 20, 89
Charles V, Emperor (Carlos I of
   Spain), 105, 123
Charles V, King of France, 93
cheddar cheese, 86–88, 90
cheese
   cheese making process, 85–92
   Egyptian cheese makers, 85
   made by medieval monks, 88–90
   noble, a catalog of, 90–92
   Roman cheese makers, 85–86